HUMAN ANA COLORING BOOK

MUSCLES
MEDICAL NOTES

50+ Unique Designs

by Delano D. Davis, M.D.

-ANATOMY & PHYSIOLOGY STUDY GUIDE-

THE MEDICAL NOTES SERIES

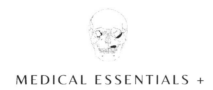

MEDICAL ESSENTIALS +

Illustrated by Delano D. Davis, M.D.
Award Winning Researcher, Tutor, and Medical Illustrator

ISBN: 9798352278376

Copyright © "Medical Essentials Plus" 2022. All Rights Reserved.

All rights reserved. This book is only for personal use. No part of this book may be copied, reproduced or distributed without written permission from the owner. Medical Essentials Plus owns the rights to this product.

Disclaimer Notice:

The information contained within this book is for educational and entertainment purposes only. The reader acknowledges that the author is not engaged in the rendering of legal, financial, medical, or professional advice. Be sure to consult a licensed professional before attempting to perform any technique described in this book.

By reading this, the reader agrees that the author is not responsible for any losses that may incur as a result of the use of the information contained within this document.

For questions and customer service;
Send us an email at medicalessentialsplus@gmail.com
Follow Us on Instagram @ medicalessentialsplus
Subscribe to our Youtube channel " Medical Essentials Plus"
for tutorials and Quizzes.

Connect with Us

Scan QR code to visit ➡

Medical Essentials Plus - Amazon Author Page

Visit our Author page to check out our wide range of atlases, and coloring workbooks on the human anatomy and physiology. We also have beautiful notebooks. Find books on;

- Gross Anatomy
- Anatomy and Physiology
- Musculoskeletal System
- Neuroanatomy
- Cardiovascular System Anatomy
- Anatomy notebooks, Journals and more

Scan QR code to visit ➡

Medical Essentials Plus - YouTube Channel

Visit the medical Essentials Plus Youtube channel and subscribe to get the tutorials and quizzes on:

- Anatomy and Physiology
- Gross Anatomy
- Clinical Medicine
- Clinical Procedures & more

Test your knowledge by taking our quizzes.

Contents

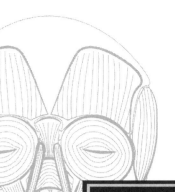

CHAPTER 1 - INTRODUCTION 7
- The Anatomical Position & Planes — 8
- Muscle Features — 9
- Types of Muscle Shapes — 18
- Skeletal Muscles - Overview — 13
- Review — 19

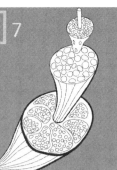

CHAPTER 2 - HEAD 21
- Facial Muscles — 23
- Facial Muscle Groups — 29
- Muscles of Mastication — 33
- Extrinsic Muscles of the Eyes — 39
- Review — 41

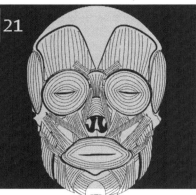

CHAPTER 3 - NECK 43
- Lateral Neck-Scalene Muscles — 45
- Anterior Neck Muscles — 47
- Deep Neck Muscles — 49
- Superficial Neck Muscles — 53
- Posterior Head and Neck — 57
- Review — 61

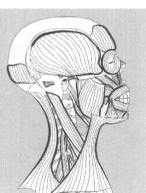

CHAPTER 4 - UPPER LIMB 63
- Hand- (Thenar Eminence) — 65
- Hand- (Hypothenar Eminence) — 71
- Hand- Interossei — 73
- Muscles of the Arm — 75
- Rotator Cuff — 77
- Muscles of the Forearm — 79
- Review — 91

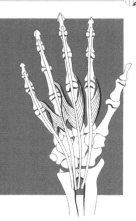

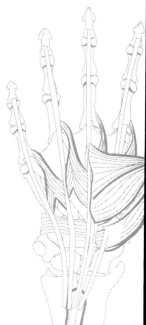

Contents

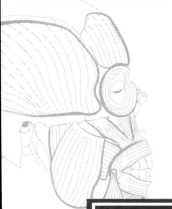

CHAPTER 5 - TRUNK   93

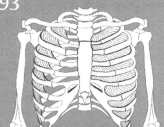

- Ribcage Muscles ---------------------------- 95
- Diaphragm ---------------------------------- 105
- Abdominal Muscles ------------------------- 107
- Trunk- Review ------------------------------ 117
- Muscles of the Back ----------------------- 119
- Muscles of the Back - Review ------------ 129

CHAPTER 6 - HIP & LOWER LIMB   131

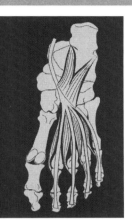

- Thigh Flexors ------------------------------------ 133
- Thigh Adductors --------------------------------- 135
- Hamstring Muscles ------------------------------ 141
- Leg Muscles -------------------------------------- 143
- Muscles of the Foot ---------------------------- 149
- Review -- 157

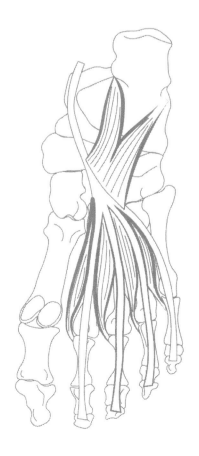

Preface

This book is a collection of unique line drawing diagrams of the human musculoskeletal system. It is the digitized version of sketches done while I was in medical school. It is designed to be used as a supplemental study guide to aid students of anatomy and physiology, and others in the healthcare field.

It should be used to aid in the visual orientation and basic identification of the structures of the human musculoskeletal system. From my own experience, learning the human anatomy can present many challenges, so preparing simple line diagrams and coloring them was a good strategy that proved to be quite useful. This practice improved my understanding, retention and recall of core concepts.

The focus is squarely placed on the identification of muscles and so little to no ligaments, no attachments, or information on origin, insertion, or nerve supply were added. The detailed coverage of the bones featured in this book can be found in book one (1) "Human Anatomy Coloring Book: Bones". It is the foundation for a series of books that breaks down the human anatomy in a layered manner, looking at each system individually but not exclusively of each other. We recommend getting book one.

Each diagram in this book is labeled with numbers and or letters and structures are identified by using the key list provided. Color coding is done by matching the number or letter of each structure with its corresponding terminology and color swatch in the Key. This will help you to quickly reference each labeled part when reviewing your work. However, there will be structures that cannot be colored in completely, such as bony landmarks, in this case, we recommend the use of a standard color in the swatch, for example. Gray.

We have included a number of review pages to help promote self-testing. Self-testing promotes content retention and evaluates understanding of the topic covered. Each review page has a diagram that should be labeled and colored, feel free to add your own notes and anotations.

Features:
-Anatomy Flash Card style format
-Pages with Diagrams and space to jot done important notes.
-Self-test review pages at the end of each chapter.
-Notes pages
-Summaries
-Quick access to our video quizzes

Stay tuned for our books on Neuroanatomy, the Digestive system, the Cardiovascular system, and more. Coloring is an easy and fun way to learn anatomy and physiology. We here at Medical Essentials Plus hope that this book will not only provide entertainment value but also play a valuable role as an educational supplement to the course material for anatomy and physiology students everywhere.

Delano D. Davis, M.D.

CHAPTER I

INTRODUCTION

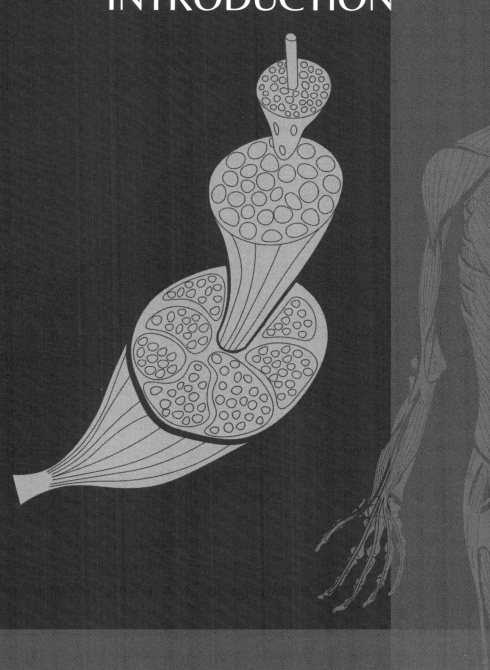
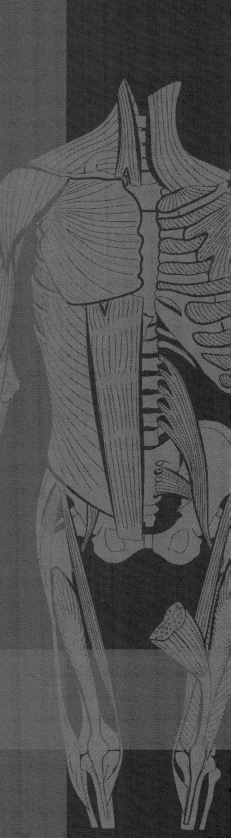

Anatomical Position & Planes — INTRODUCTION

ANATOMICAL POSITION

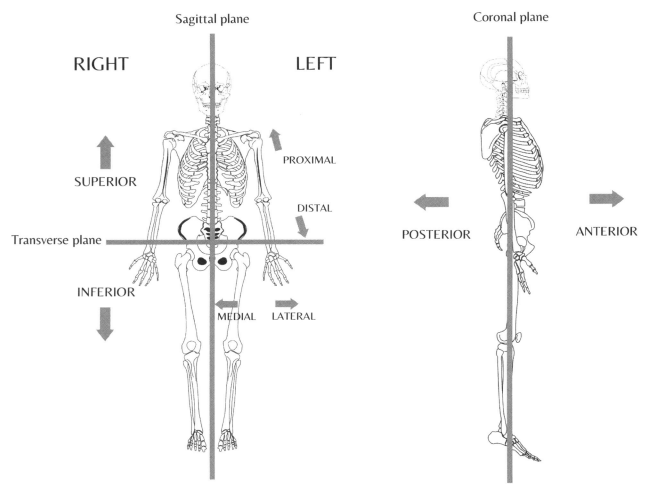

The anatomical position is represented when a subject's body is standing erect, head and eyes are in a forward position, and both arms are at the sides with palms facing forward. The legs are together with the toes pointing forward.

PLANES

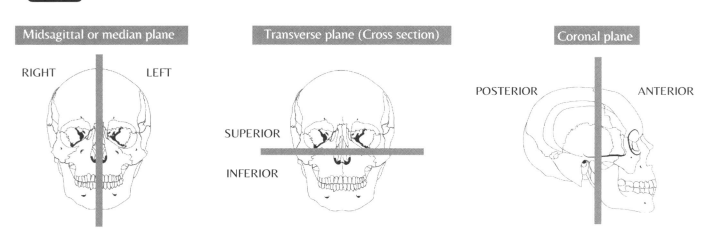

Muscle Features — INTRODUCTION

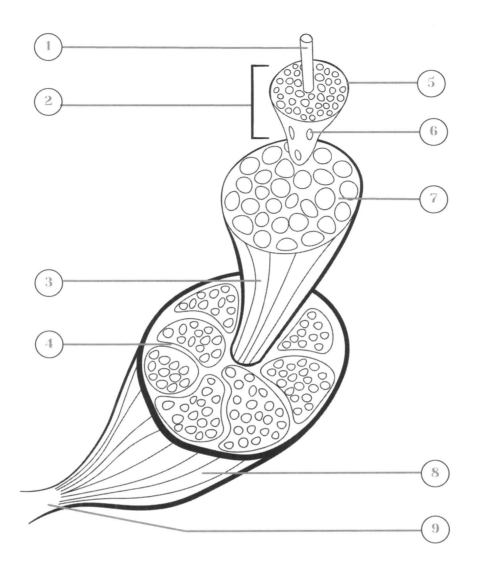

1. Myofibril
2. Muscle Fiber (Multinucleated Cell)
3. Fascicle
4. Perimysium (Wraps fascicle)
5. Sarcolemma
6. Nucleus
7. Endomysium (Wraps muscle fiber)
8. Epimysium (Wraps whole muscle)
9. Tendon (Attach to bone)

NOTES

Types of Muscle Shapes

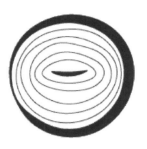
CIRCULAR MUSCLE

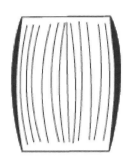
PARALLEL MUSCLE (RECTANGULAR)

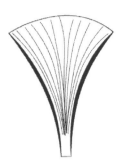
CONVERGENT/ TRIANGULARM USCLE

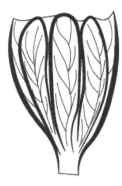
PENNATE MUSCLE (MULTIPENNATE)

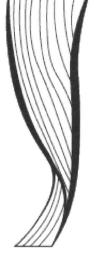
SPIRAL MUSCLE

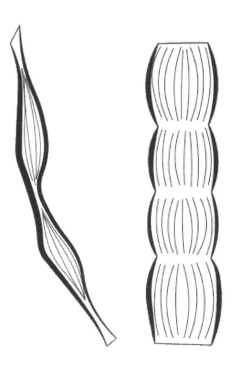
BIVENTER MUSCLE

PARALLEL MUSCLE (STRAPLIKE WITH TENDINOUS INTERRUPTIONS)

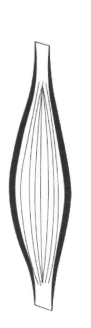
PARALLEL MUSCLE (FUSIFORM)

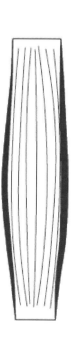
PARALLEL MUSCLE (STRAPLIKE)

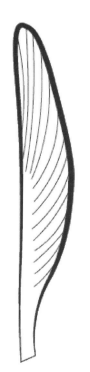
PENNATE MUSCLE (UNIPENNATE)

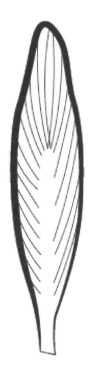
PENNATE MUSCLE (BIPENNATE)

Types of Muscle Shapes

INTRODUCTION

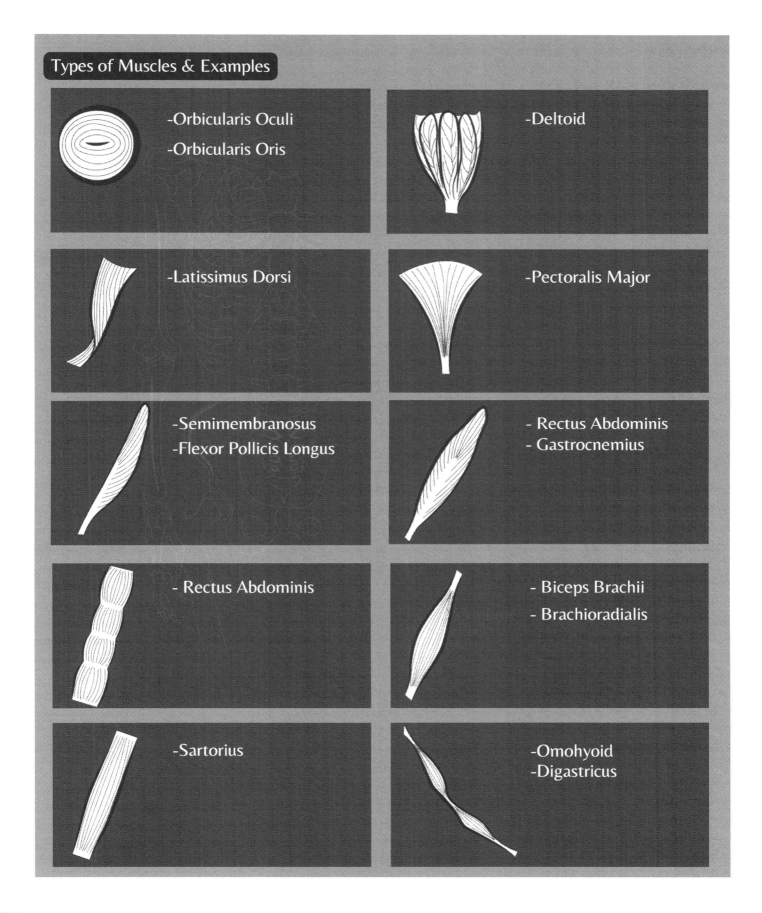

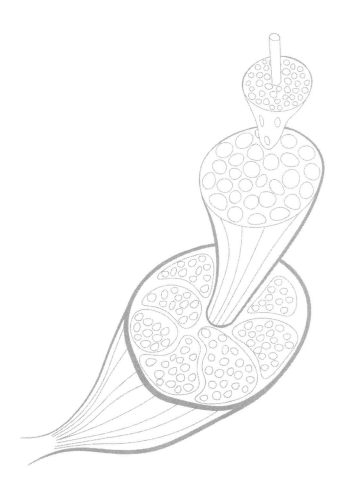

Skeletal Muscles: Overview

INTRODUCTION

Anterior view

1. Trapezius
2. Deltoid
3. Pectoral Major
4. Biceps Brachii
5. External Oblique
6. Rectus Abdominis
7. Tensor Fasciae Latae
8. Vastus Intermedius
9. Platysma
10. Coracobrachialis
11. Pectoral Minor
12. Internal Intercostal
13. Psoas Major
14. Piriformis
15. Sartorius
16. Rectus Femoris
17. Vastus Lateralis
18. Vastus Medialis

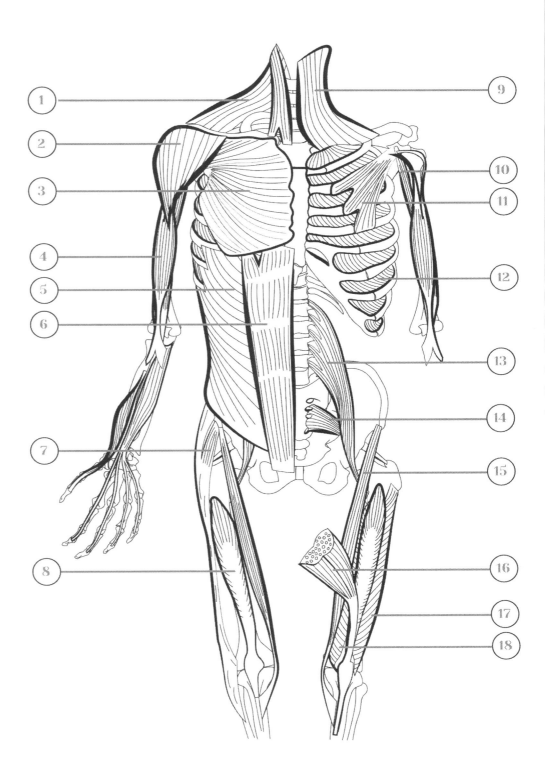

INTRODUCTION

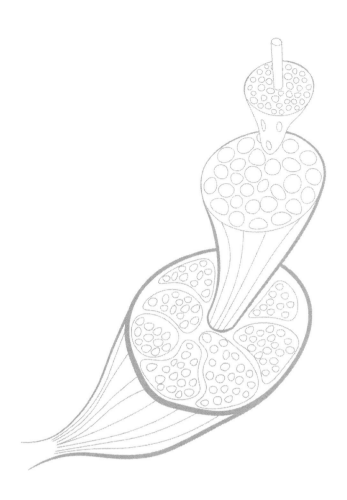

Skeletal Muscles: Overview

INTRODUCTION

Posterior view

1. Trapezius
2. Deltoid
3. Latissimus Dorsi
4. Gluteus Minimus
5. Quadratus Femoris
6. Rectus Abdominis
7. Gracilis
8. Levator Scapulae
9. Supraspinatus
10. Teres Major
11. Triceps Brachii
12. Serratus Posterior Inferior
13. Gluteus Maximus
14. Semimembranosus
15. Biceps Femoris

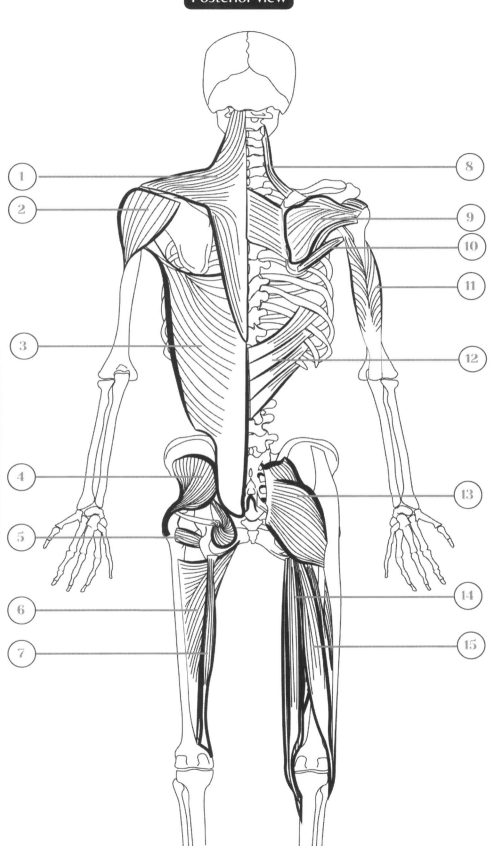

INTRODUCTION

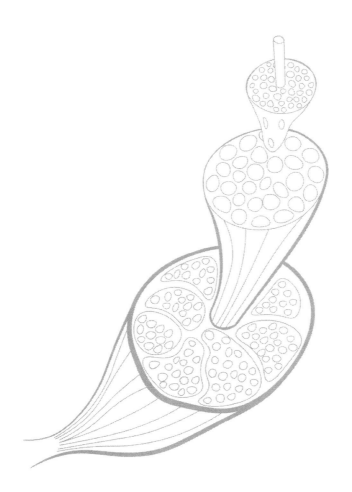

Skeletal Muscles: Overview

INTRODUCTION

Lateral view

1. Deltoid
2. Gluteus Maximus
3. Biceps Femoris
4. Gastrocnemius
5. Serratus Anterior
6. Internal Oblique
7. Tensor Fasciae Latae
8. Rectus Femoris
9. Tibialis Anterior

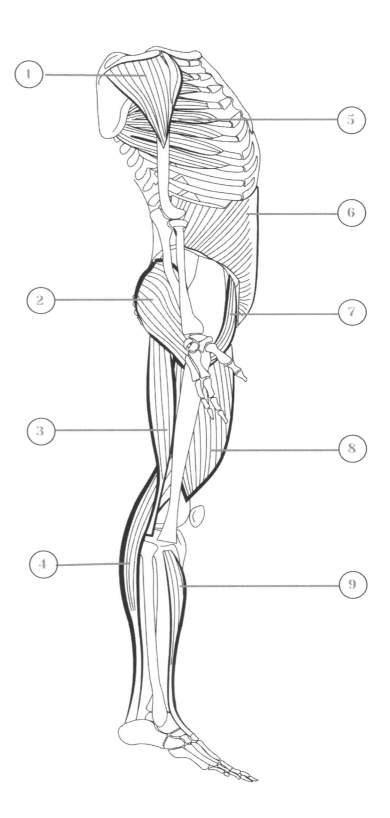

INTRODUCTION

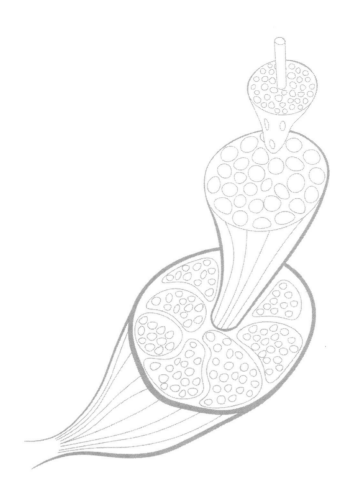

Review

INTRODUCTION

Posterior view

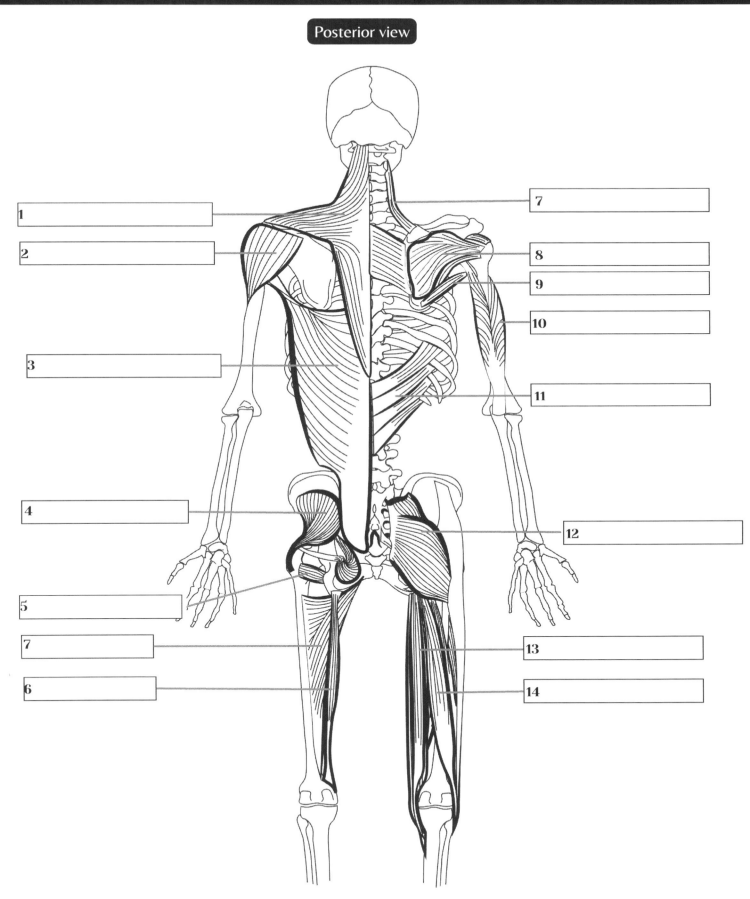

1.
2.
3.
4.
5.
7.
6.
7.
8.
9.
10.
11.
12.
13.
14.

INTRODUCTION

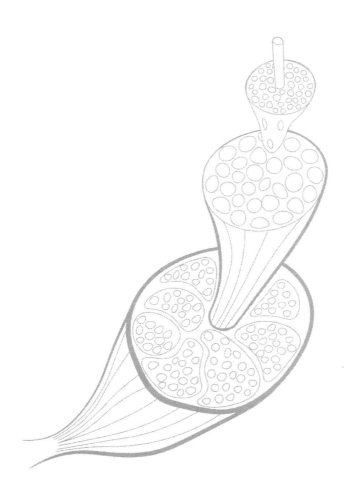

CHAPTER II

HEAD

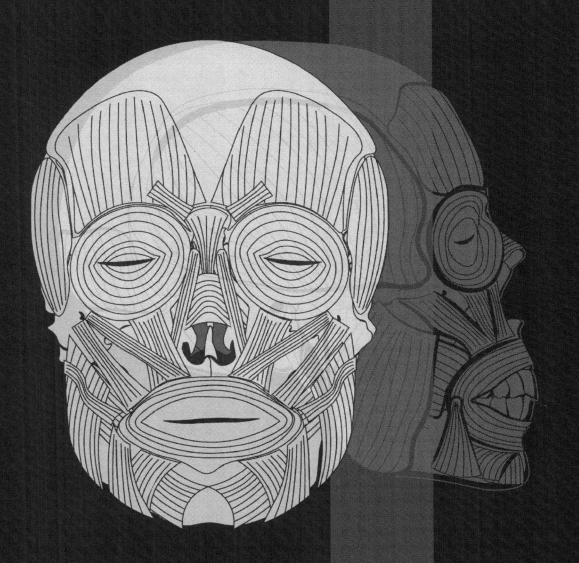

The Muscles of Head and Face

Muscles and their functions:

- Occipitalis: Pulls the scalp backwards.
- Frontalis: Wrinkles the forehead and lifts eyebrows.
- Orbicularis Oculi (Orbital and Palpebral parts) : Closes eyelids
- Corrugator supercilii: Wrinkles the skin between the eyebrows.
- Zygomaticus Major: Lifts the upper lip.
- Buccinator: Contracts the cheeks
- Risorius: Retracts the angle of the mouth. Produces a smile.
- Mentalis: Depresses the lower lip and wrinkles the skin of the chin.
- Platysma: Depresses lower lip and wrinkles the neck skin
- Depressor anguli oris: Depresses the lower lip
- Levator Anguli Oris: Elevates the upper lip into a smile
- Levator labii superioris aleaque nasi: Elevates the upper lip and flares the nostrils.
- Procerus: Draws down medial part of eyebrow and wrinkles nose.

Facial Muscles - Anterior view

HEAD

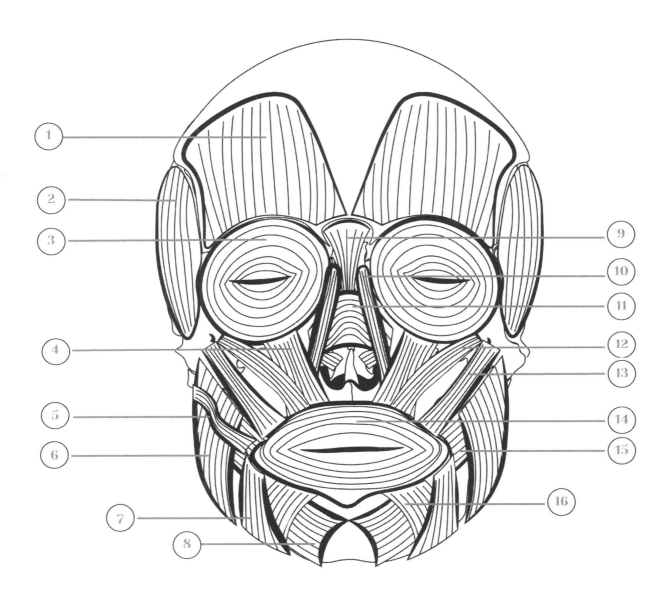

- 1. Frontalis
- 2. Temporalis
- 3. Orbicularis Oculi
- 4. Levator Labii Superioris
- 5. Risorius
- 6. Masseter
- 7. Depressor Anguli Oris
- 8. Mentalis
- 9. Procerus
- 10. Levator Labii Superioris Alaeque Nasi
- 11. Nasalis
- 12. Zygomaticus Minor
- 13. Zygomaticus Major
- 14. Orbicularis Oris
- 15. Buccinator
- 16. Depressor Labii Inferioris

NOTES

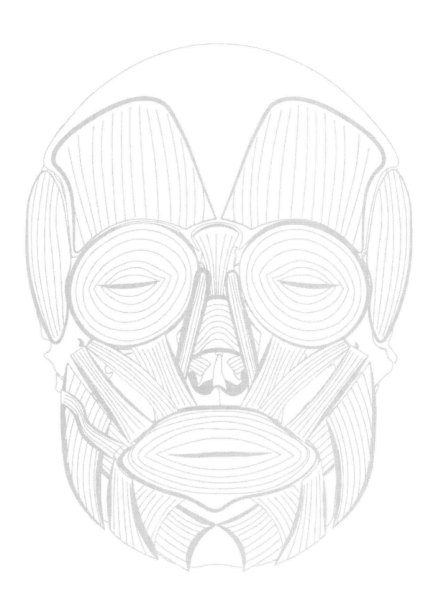

Facial Muscles - Lateral View

HEAD

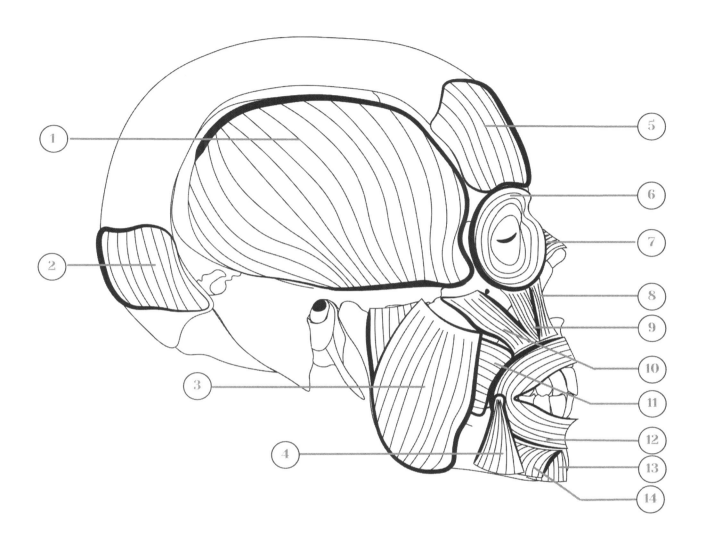

1. Temporalis
2. Occipitalis
3. Masseter
4. Depressor Anguli Oris
5. Frontalis
6. Orbicularis Oculi
7. Nasalis
8. Levator Labii Superioris
9. Zygomaticus Minor
10. Zygomaticus Minor
11. Buccinator
12. Orbicularis Oris
13. Mentalis
14. Depressor Labii Inferioris

NOTES

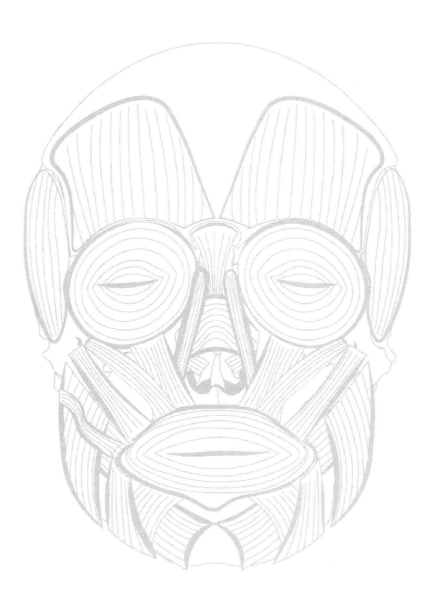

Facial Muscles - Lateral View

HEAD

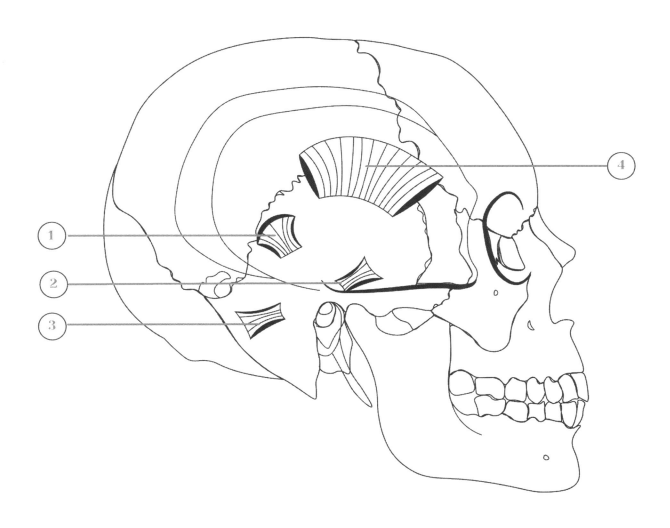

1. Auricularis Superior
2. Auricularis Anterior
3. Auricularis Posterior
4. Temporoparietalis

NOTES

HEAD

Facial Muscles - Oral Group

HEAD

Oral group

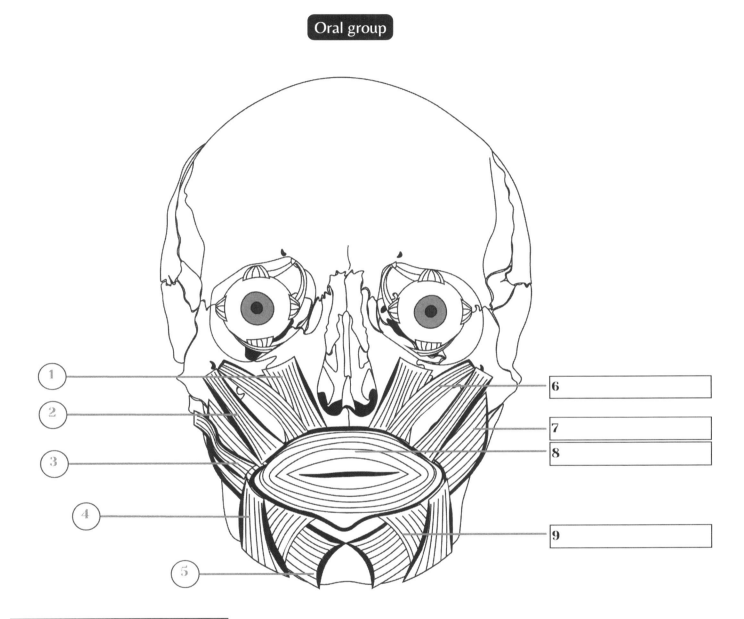

- 1. Levator Labii Superioris
- 2. Zygomaticus Major
- 3. Risorius
- 4. Depressor Anguli Oris
- 5. Mentalis
- 6. Zygomaticus Minor
- 7. Buccinator
- 8. Orbicularis Oris
- 9. Depressor Labii Inferioris

NOTES

HEAD

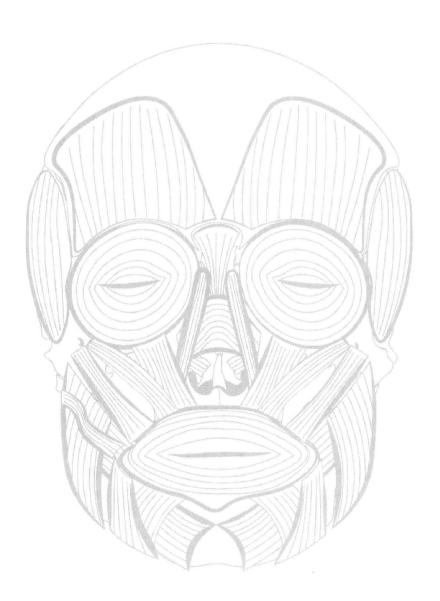

Facial Muscle Groups

HEAD

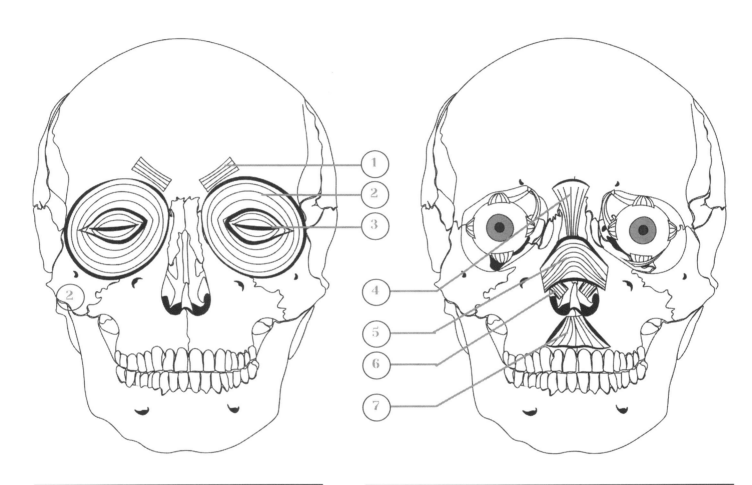

Orbital group

- 1. Corrugator Supercilii
- 2. Orbicularis Oculi (Orbital part)
- 3. Orbicularis Oculi (Palpebral part)

Nasal group

- 4. Procerus
- 5. Nasalis (Transverse/ Compressor Naris)
- 6. Nasalis (Alar/ Dilator Naris Posterior)
- 7. Depressor Nasi Septi

NOTES

The Muscles of Mastication

The muscles of mastication can be divided into the primary muscles and secondary or accessory muscles.

The primary muscles include:

- Masseter: Clenches teeth, Closes the lower jaw.
- Temporalis:
- Lateral pterygoid
- Medial pterygoid: Closes the lower jaw, clenches teeth

The secondary muscles include:

Suprahyoid muscles
- Buccinator
- Digastricus
- Geniohyoid
- Mylohyoid

Infrahyoid muscles
- Omohyoid
- thyrohyoid
- Sternohyoid
- Sternothyroid

Muscles of Mastication
HEAD

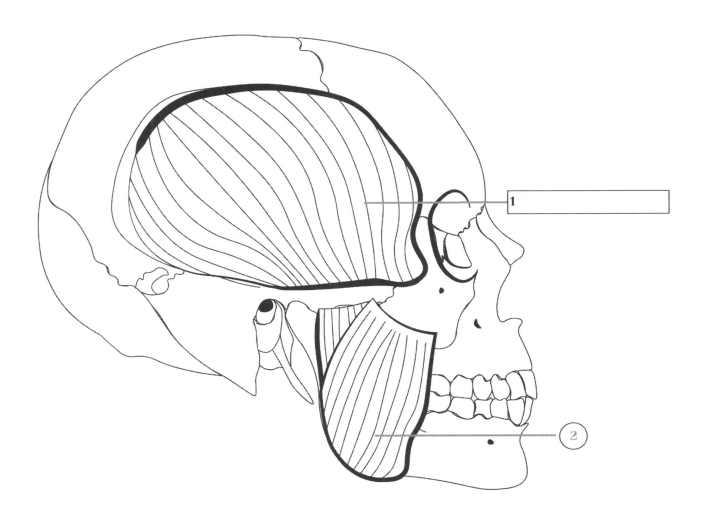

1. Temporalis
2. Masseter

NOTES

HEAD

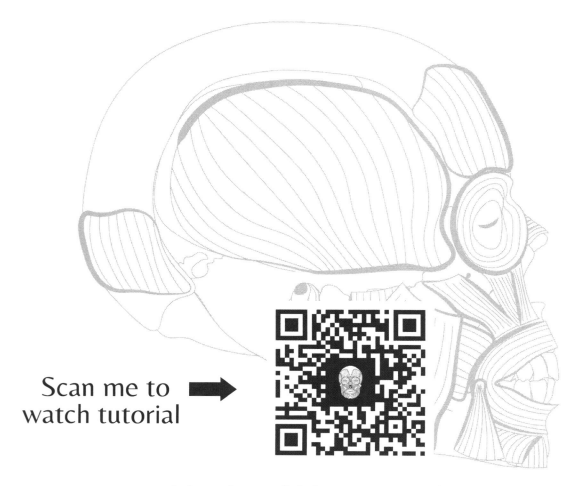

Scan me to watch tutorial ➡

Muscles of Mastication Anatomy and Physiology Tutorial.

Overview of all four (4) Muscles:
- Origin
- Insertion
- Innervation
- Action

Muscles of Mastication

HEAD

Pterygoid muscles (Lateral view)

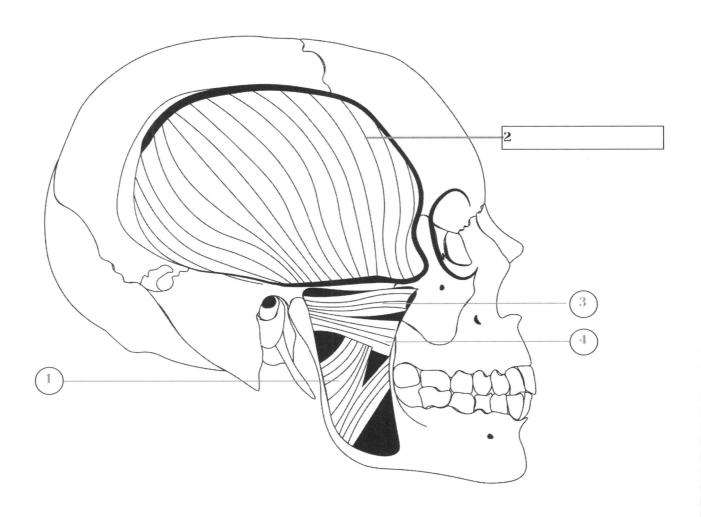

- 1. Medial Pterygoid (Pterygoideus Medialis)
- 2. Temporalis
- 3. Lateral pterygoid (Pterygoideus Lateralis- Superior head)
- 4. Lateral pterygoid (Pterygoideus Lateralis- Inferior head)

NOTES

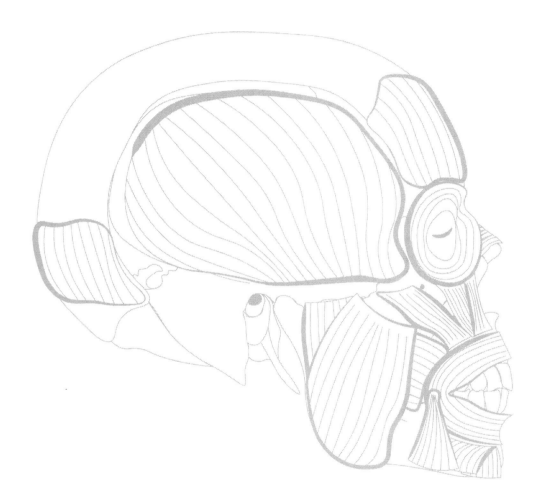

Muscles of Mastication — HEAD

Pterygoid muscles (Posterior view)

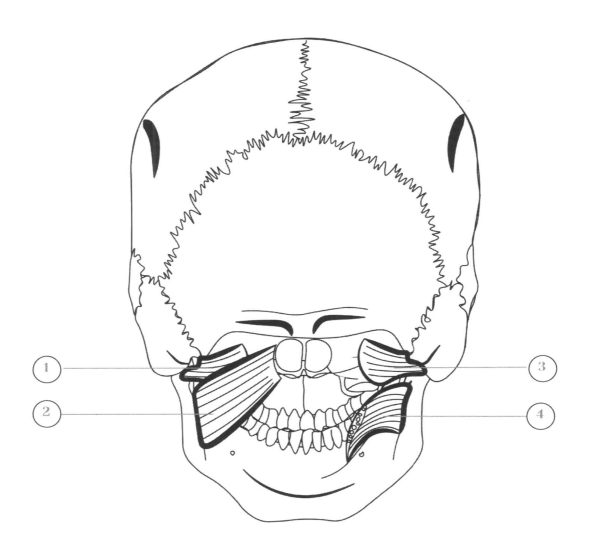

- 1. Left lateral pterygoid
- 2. Left medial Pterygoid
- 3. Right lateral pterygoid
- 4. Right Medial pterygoid (Cut)

NOTES

HEAD

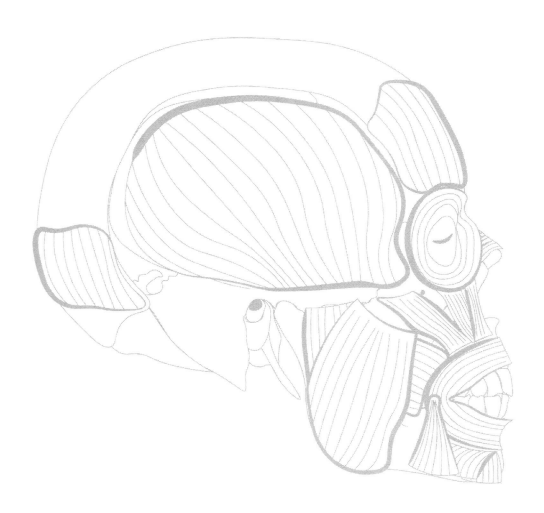

Extrinsic Muscles of the Eye

HEAD

(lateral view)

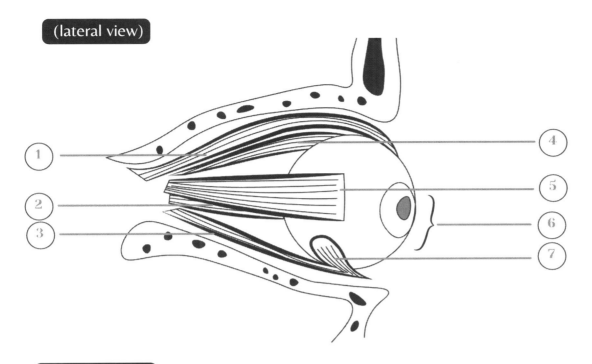

(Anterior view)

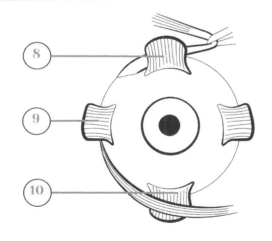
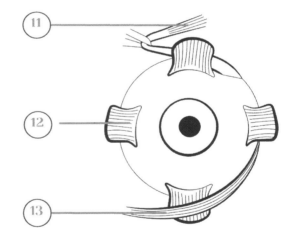

1. Superior oblique
2. Medial rectus
3. Inferior rectus
4. Superior rectus
5. Lateral rectus
6. Eyeball
7. Inferior oblique
8. Superior rectus
9. Lateral rectus
10. Inferior rectus
11. Superior oblique
12. Medial rectus
13. Inferior oblique

NOTES

HEAD

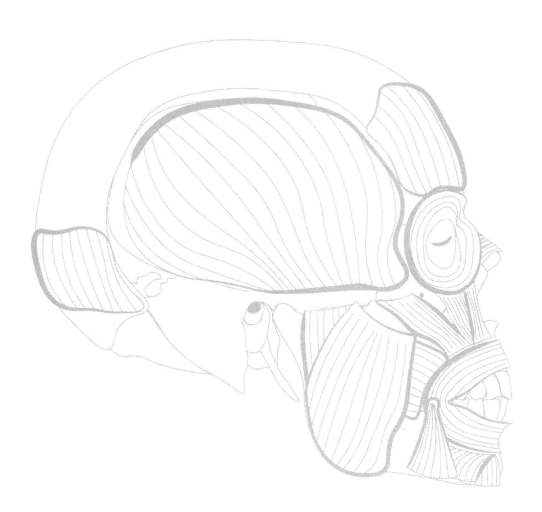

Facial Muscles - Review   HEAD

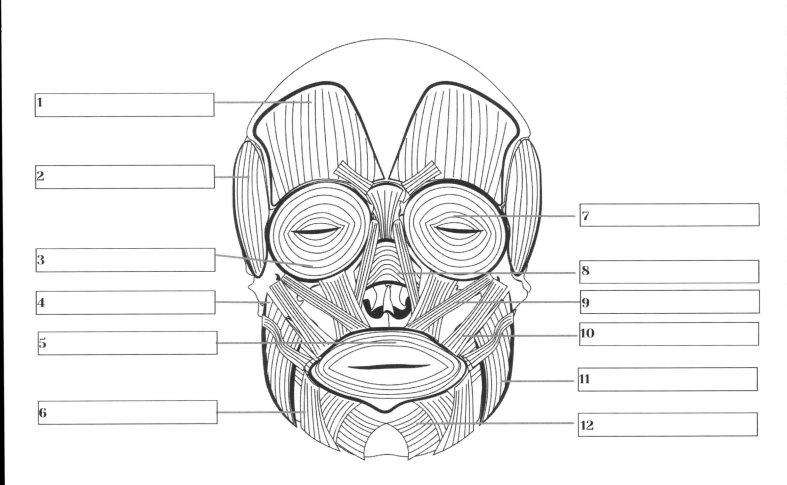

1.
2.
3.
4.
5.
6.
7.
8.
9.
10.
11.
12.

HEAD

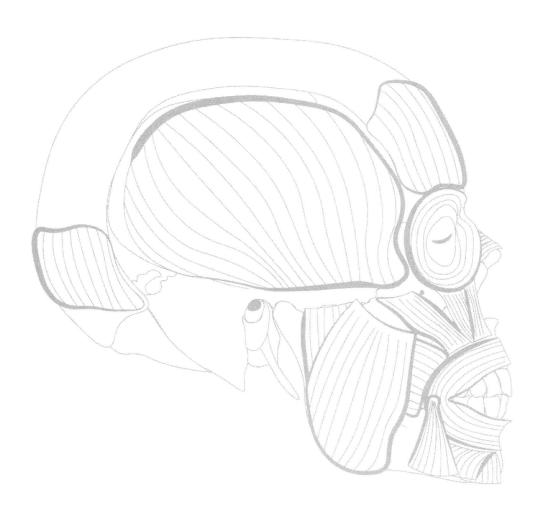

CHAPTER III

NECK

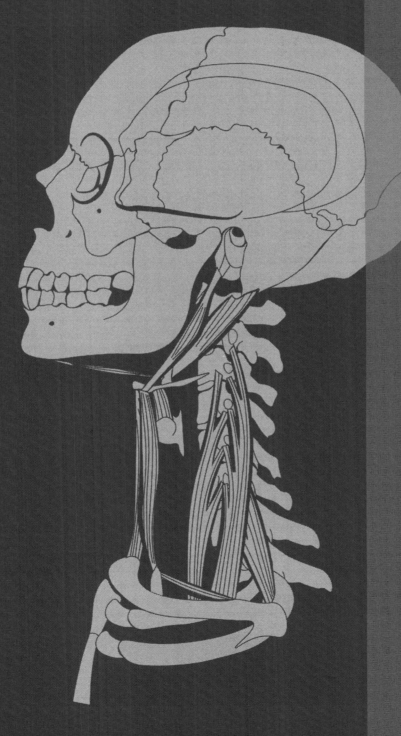

The muscles of Neck

The muscles of neck can be divided into the anterior, lateral, and posterior muscles.

The anterior muscles include:

- Superficial muscles: Platysma, sternocleidomastoid
- Suprahyoid muscles: Digastric, mylohyoid, geniohyoid, stylohyoid
- Infrahyoid muscles: Sternohyoid, sternothyroid, thyrohyoid, omohyoid
- Anterior vertebral muscles: Rectus capitis, longus capitis, longus colli

The lateral muscles:

- Scalene muscles: Anterior scalene, middle scalene, posterior scalene muscles

The posterior muscles:

- Superficial layer: Trapezius, splenius capitis, splenius cervicis
- Deep layer: Cervical transversospinales muscles (semispinalis capitis, semispinalis cervicis)
- Deepest layer: Suboccipital muscles (rectus capitis posterior major, rectus capitis posterior minor, obliquus capitis superior, obliquus capitis inferior)

Scalene Muscles

NECK

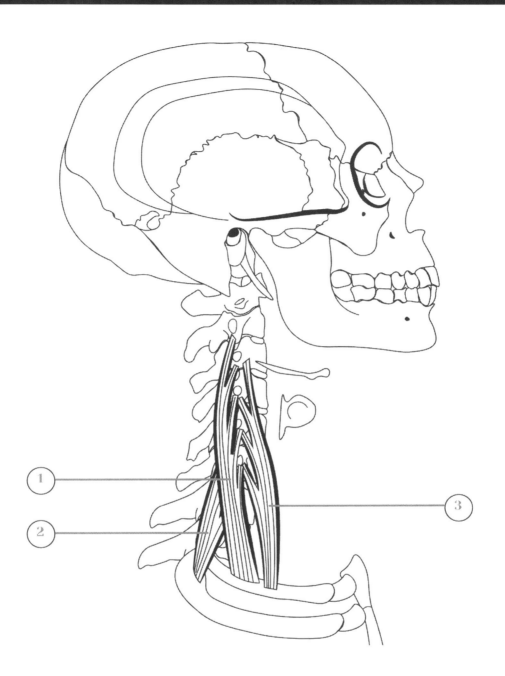

1. Scalenus Medius (Middle Scalene)
2. Scalenus Posterior (Posterior Scalene)
3. Scalenus Anterior (Anterior Scalene)

NOTES

NECK

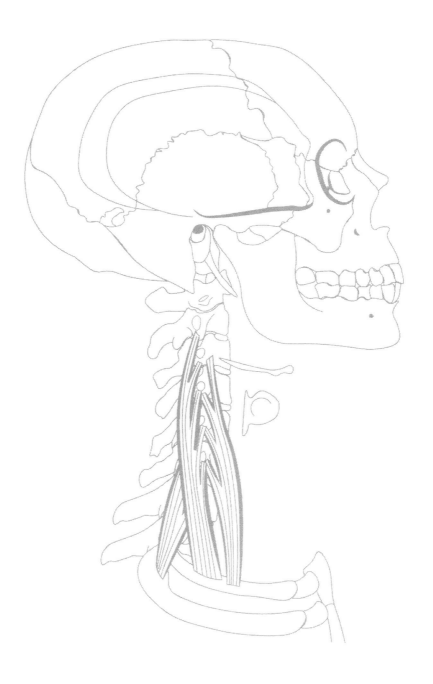

Anterior Neck Muscles

NECK

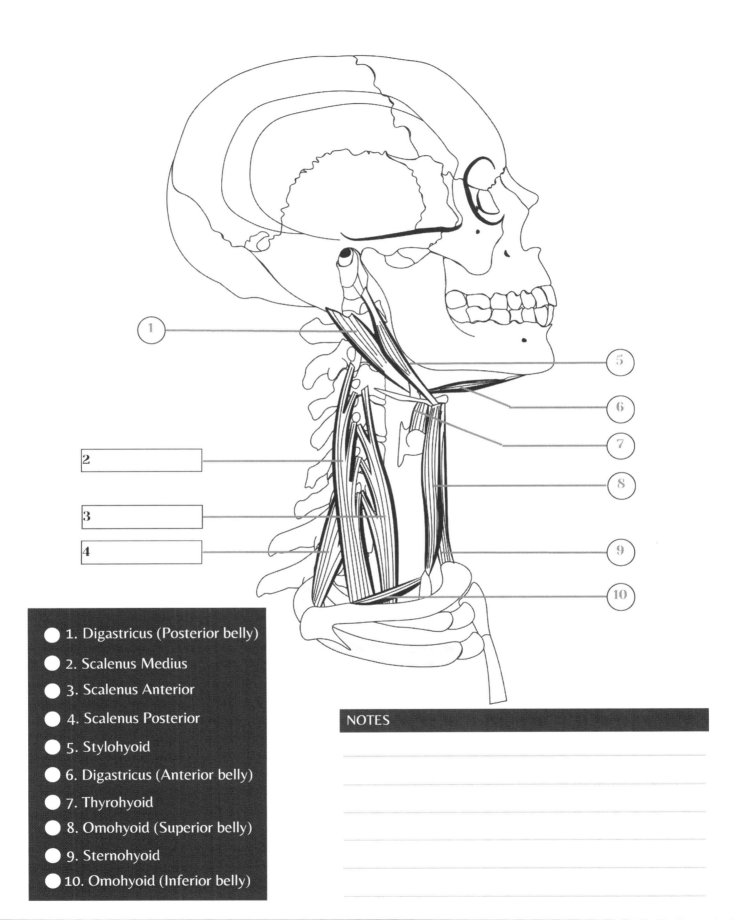

- 1. Digastricus (Posterior belly)
- 2. Scalenus Medius
- 3. Scalenus Anterior
- 4. Scalenus Posterior
- 5. Stylohyoid
- 6. Digastricus (Anterior belly)
- 7. Thyrohyoid
- 8. Omohyoid (Superior belly)
- 9. Sternohyoid
- 10. Omohyoid (Inferior belly)

NOTES

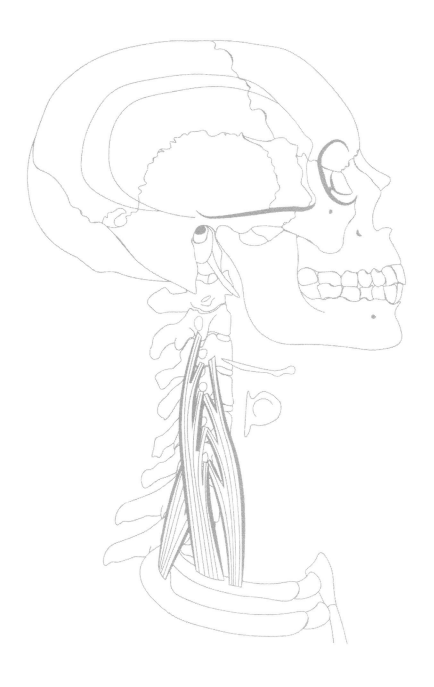

Neck Muscles (Deep) - Anterior view

NECK

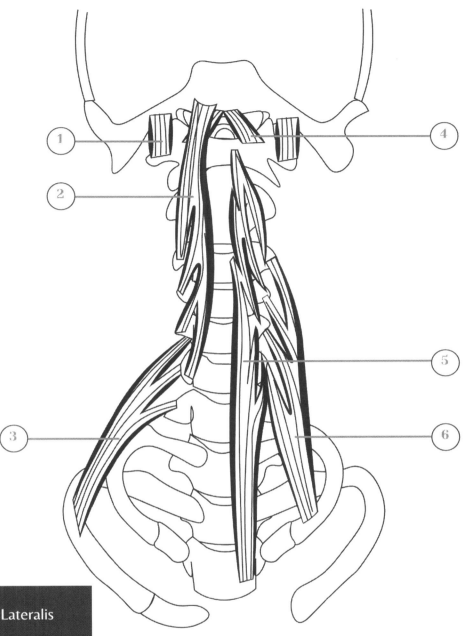

- 1. Rectus Capitis Lateralis
- 2. Longus Capitis
- 3. Scalenus Posterior
- 4. Rectus Capitis Posterior
- 5. Longus Colli
- 6. Scalenus Anterior

NOTES

NECK

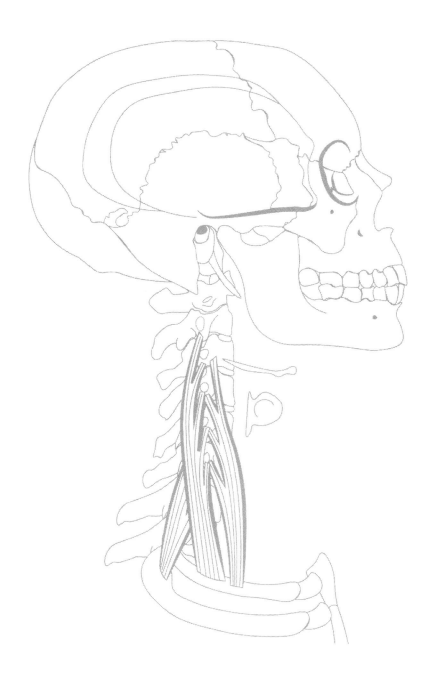

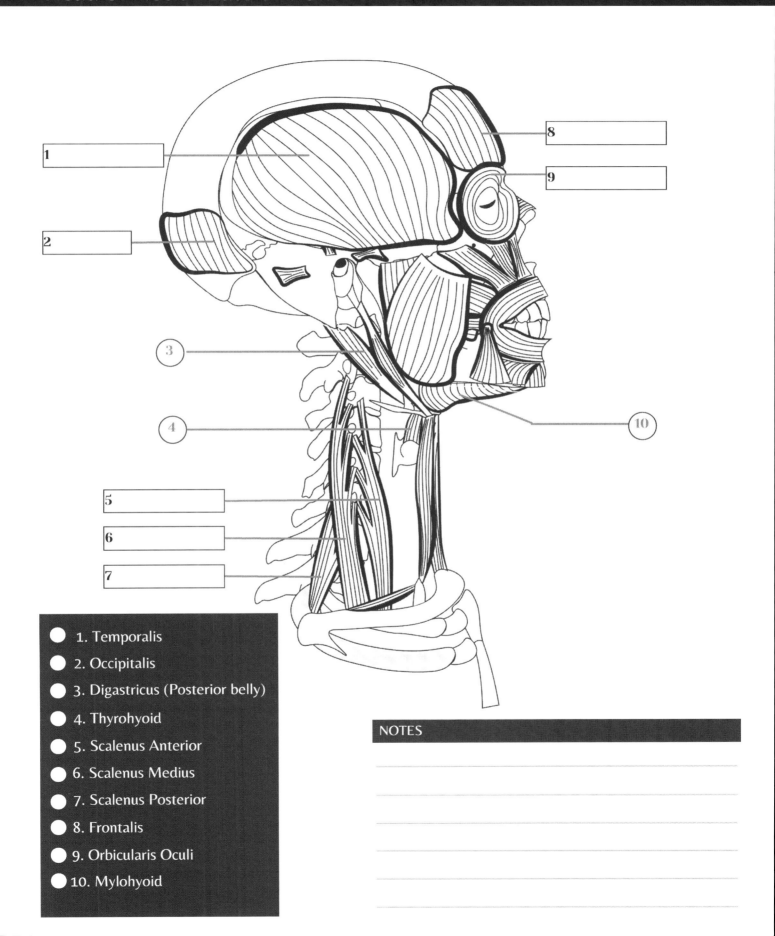

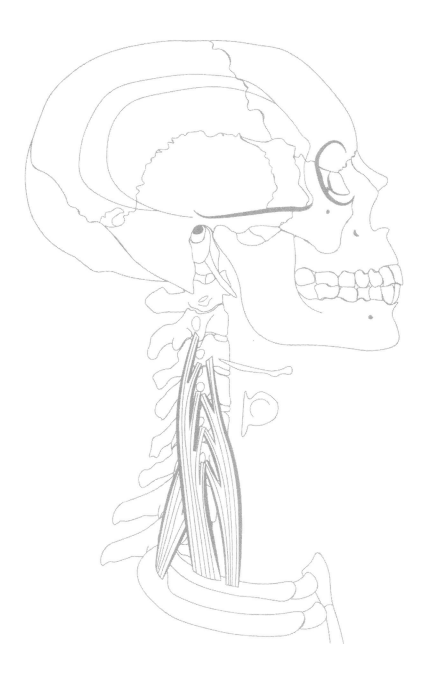

Superficial Neck Muscles

NECK

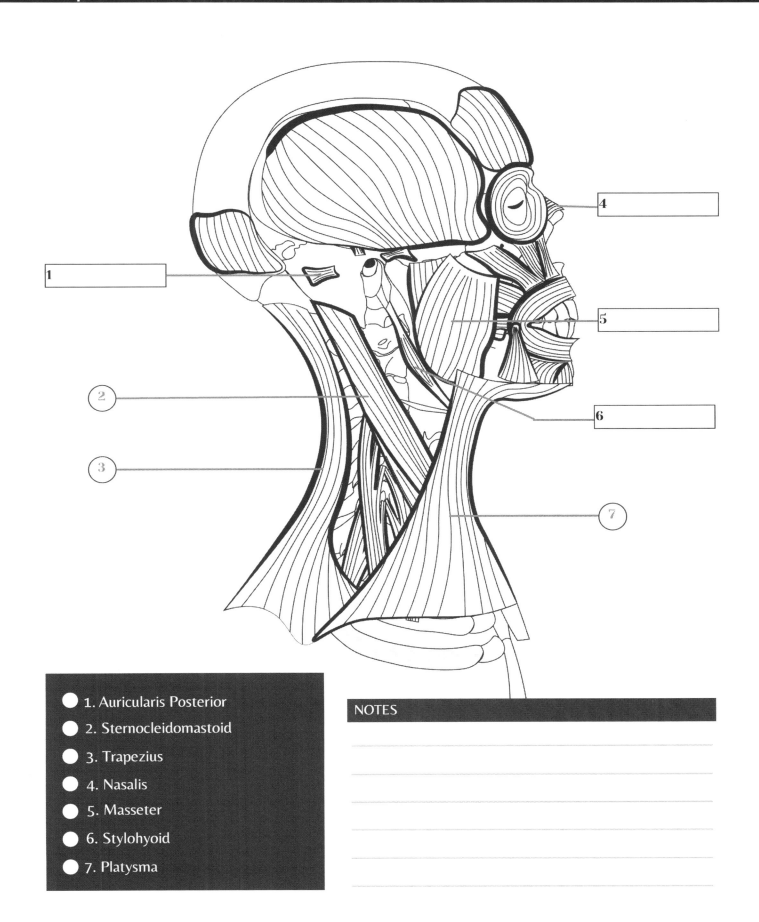

- 1. Auricularis Posterior
- 2. Sternocleidomastoid
- 3. Trapezius
- 4. Nasalis
- 5. Masseter
- 6. Stylohyoid
- 7. Platysma

NOTES

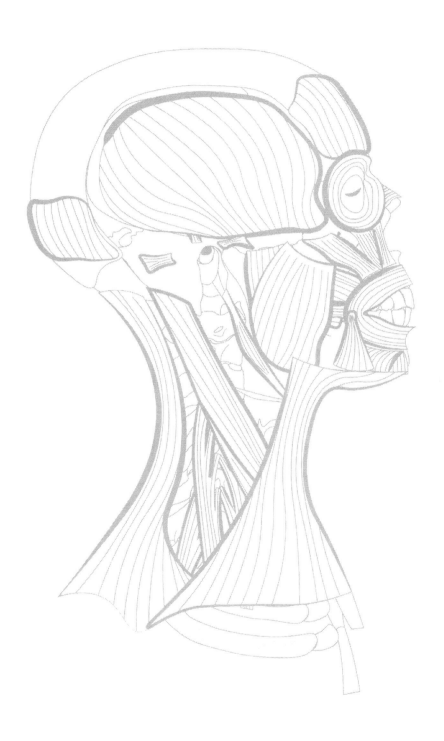

Neck Muscles (Anterior view)

NECK

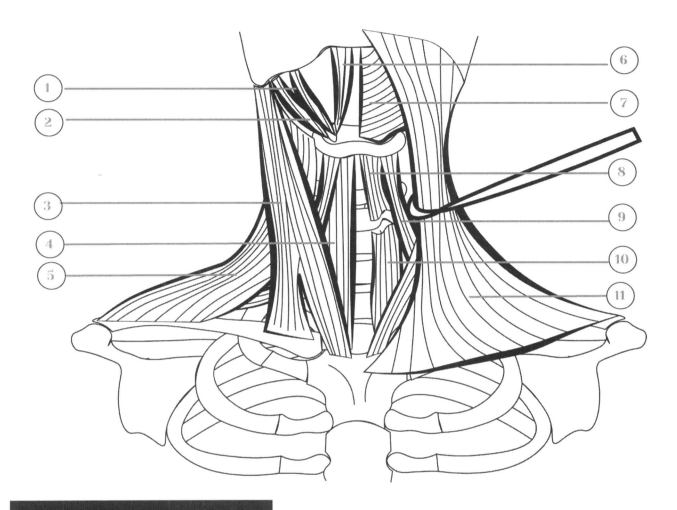

- 1. Digastricus (Posterior belly)
- 2. Stylohyoid
- 3. Sternocleidomastoid
- 4. Sternohyoid
- 5. Trapezius
- 6. Digastricus (Anterior belly)
- 7. Mylohyoid
- 8. Thyrohyoid
- 9. Omohyoid (Superior belly)
- 10. Sternothyroid
- 11. Platysma

NOTES

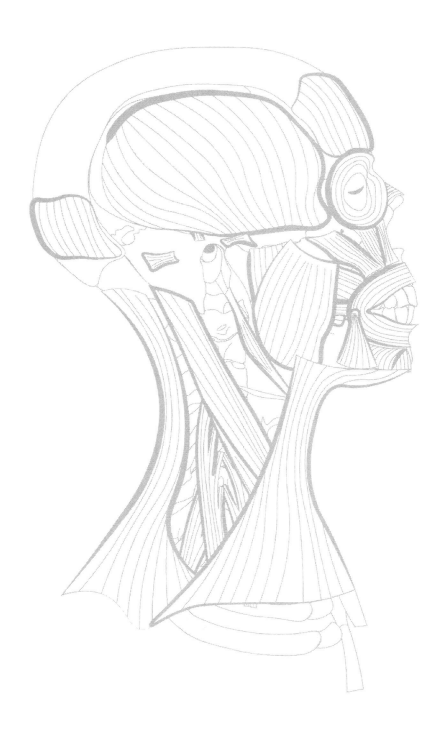

Posterior Head & Neck (Deep)

NECK

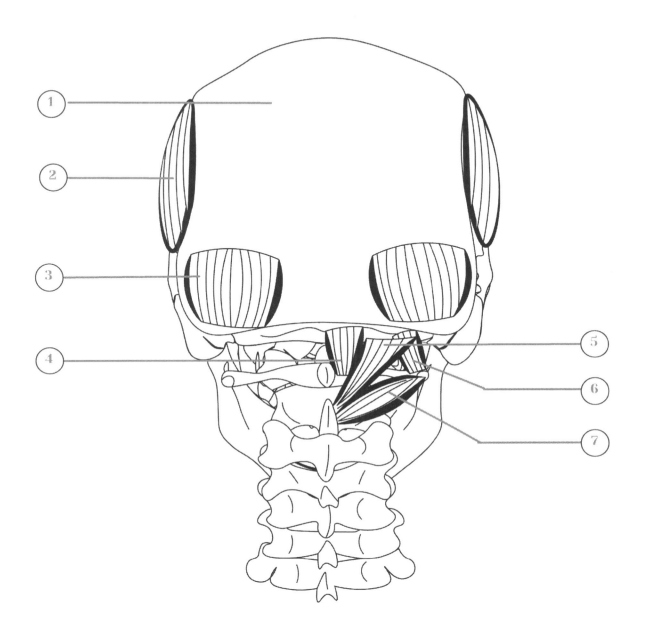

1. Epicranius
2. Temporalis
3. Occipitalis (Epicranius)
4. Rectus capitis posterior minor
5. Rectus capitis posterior major
6. Obliquus capitis superior
7. Obliquus capitis inferior

NOTES

NECK

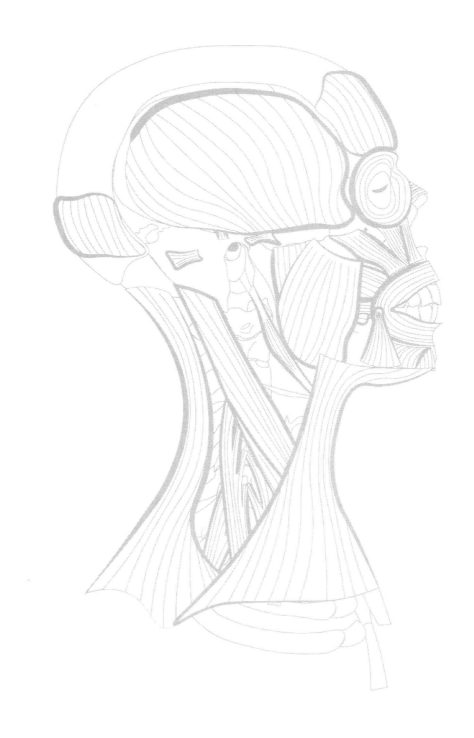

Posterior Head & Neck (Deep)

NECK

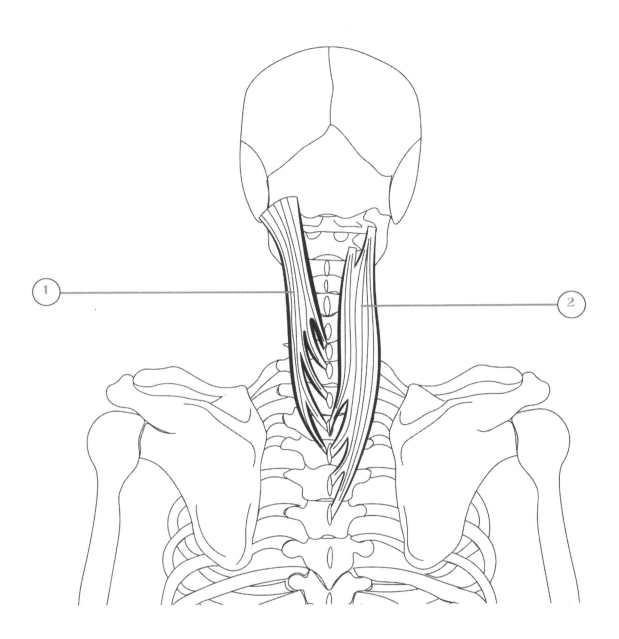

- 1. Splenius Capitis
- 2. Splenius Cervicis

NOTES

Muscle Anatomy Video Quiz

NECK

Scan me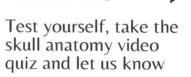

Test yourself, take the skull anatomy video quiz and let us know your score.

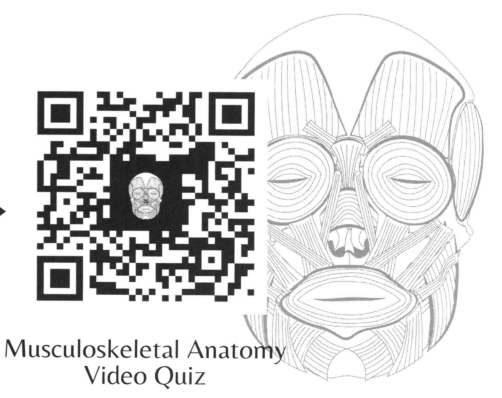

Musculoskeletal Anatomy Video Quiz

Head & Neck - Review NECK

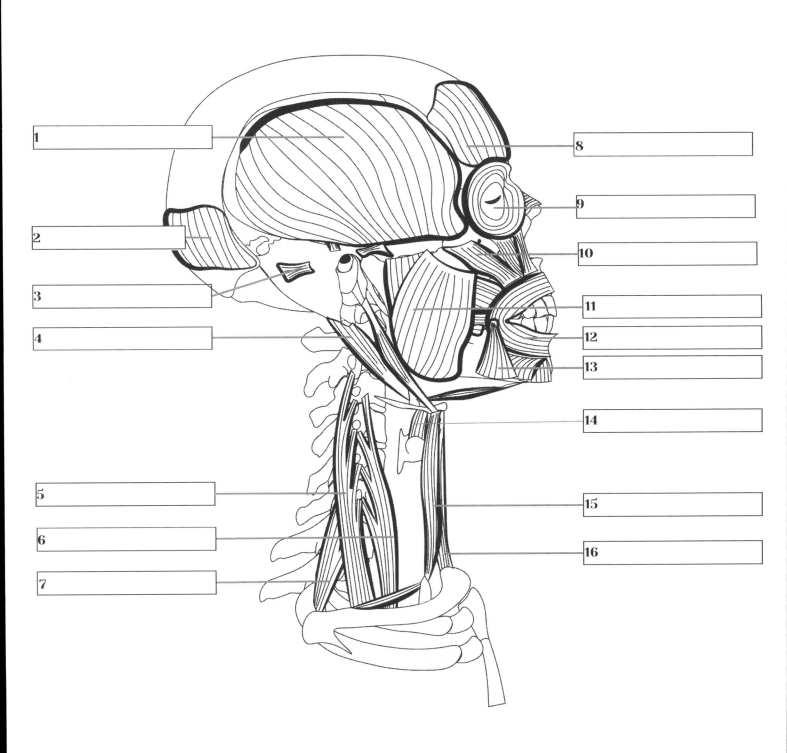

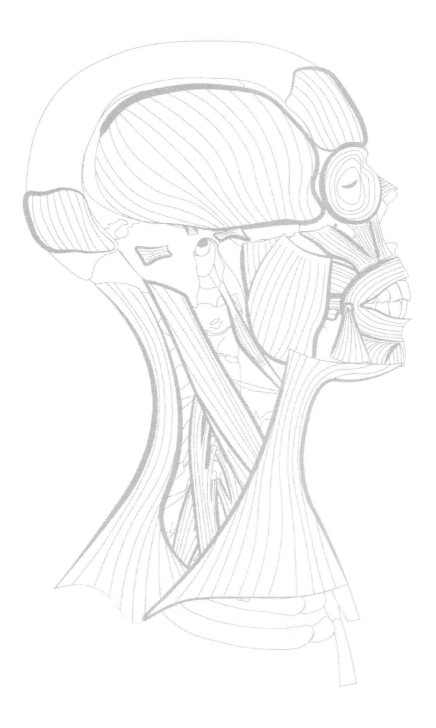

CHAPTER IV

UPPER LIMB

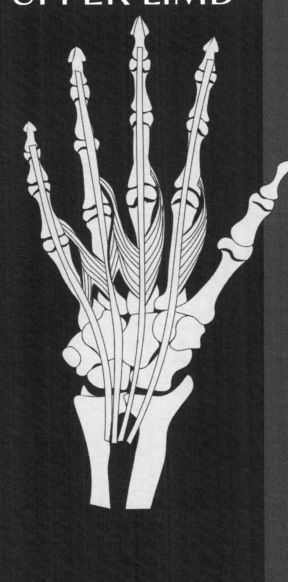

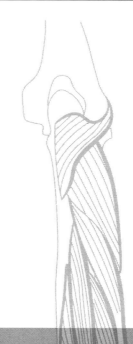

The Muscles of Hand & Wrist

The muscles of hand can be divided based on where they act.

Muscles that act on the wrist (Carpi):

- Extensor Carpi Radialis Longus
- Extensor Carpi Radialis Brevis
- Extensor Carpi Ulnaris
- Flexor Carpi Ulnaris
- Flexor Carpi Radialis
- Palmaris Longus

Intrinsic muscles that act only on the fingers (digits):

- Thenar muscles
- Adductor Pollicis
- Hyperthenar muscles
- Lumbricales
- Dorsal Interossei
- Palmar Interossei

Extrinsic Muscles of the thumb (I digit)

- Flexor Pollicis Longus
- Extensor Pollicis Longus
- Extensor Pollicis Brevis
- Abductor Pollicis Longus

Intrinsic muscles of (II- IV digits)

- Extensor Digitorum
- Extensor Indicis
- Extensor Digiti Minimi
- Flexor Digitorum Superficiales
- Flexor Digitorum Profundus

Hand - Palmar view (Thenar Eminence)

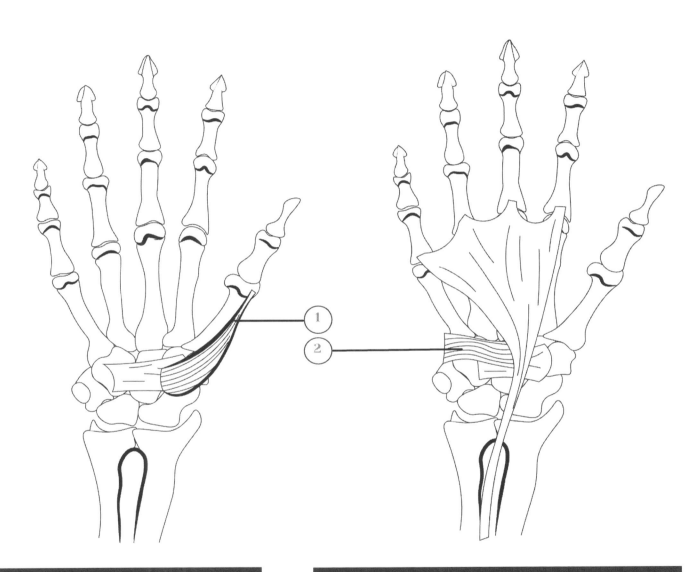

- 1. Abductor Pollicis Brevis
- 2. Palmaris Brevis

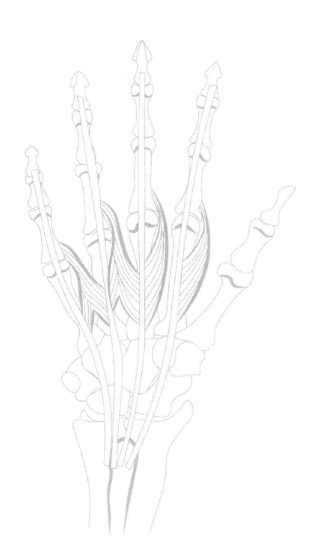

Hand - Palmar view (Thenar Eminence)

UPPER LIMB

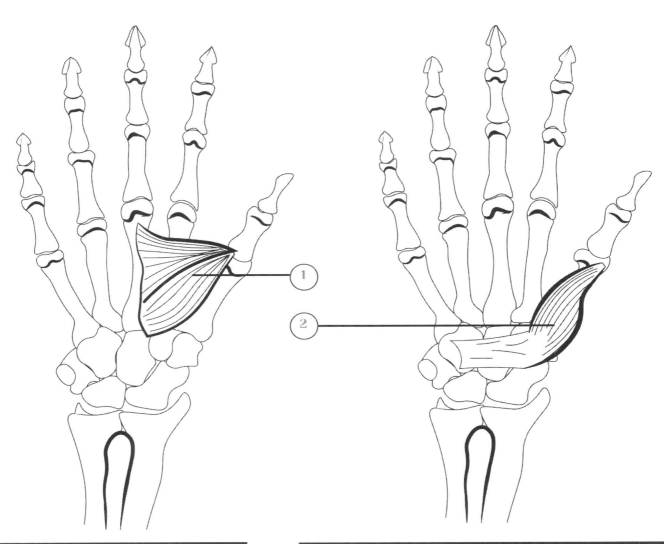

- 1. Adductor Pollicis
- 2. Opponens Pollicis

NOTES

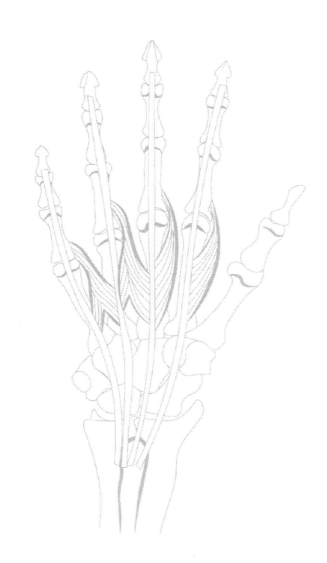

Hand - Palmar view (Thenar Eminence)

UPPER LIMB

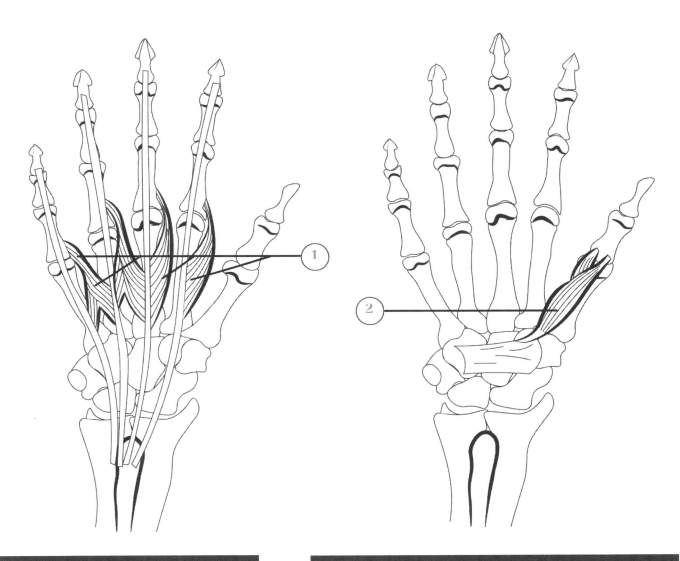

- 1. Lumbricales
- 2. Flexor Pollicis Brevis

NOTES

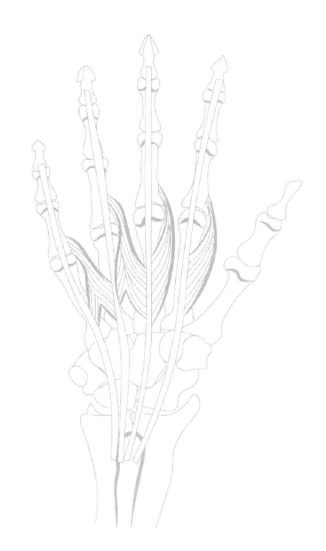

Hand - Palmar view (Hypothenar Eminence)

UPPER LIMB

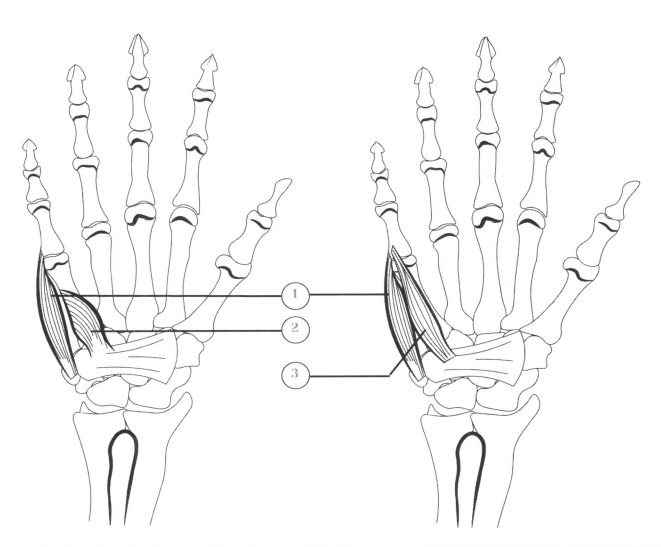

1. Abductor Digiti Minimi
2. Opponens Digiti Minimi
2. Flexor Digiti Minimi Brevis

NOTES

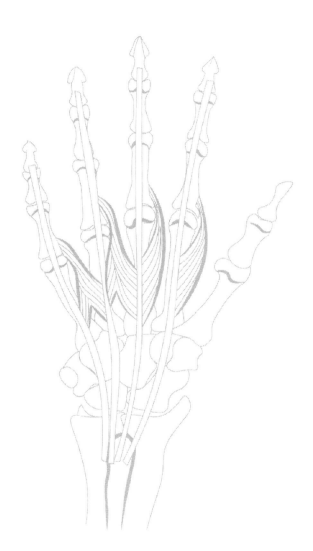

Hand - Interossei

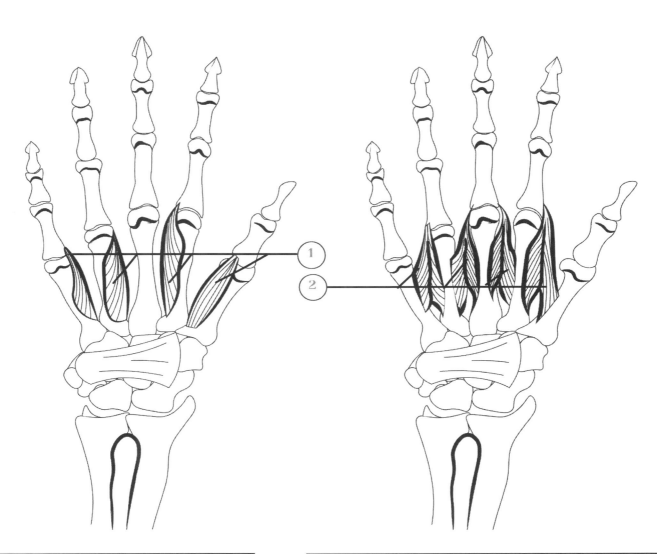

- 1. Palmar Interossei
- 2. Dorsal Interossei

NOTES

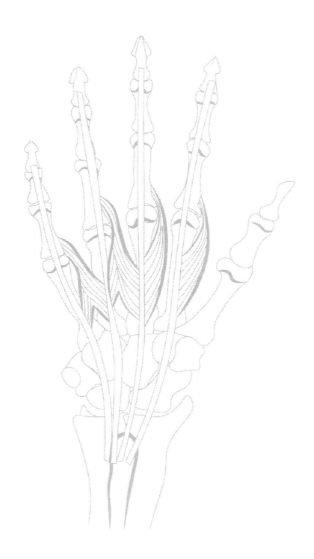

Muscles of the Arm (Anterior view)

UPPER LIMB

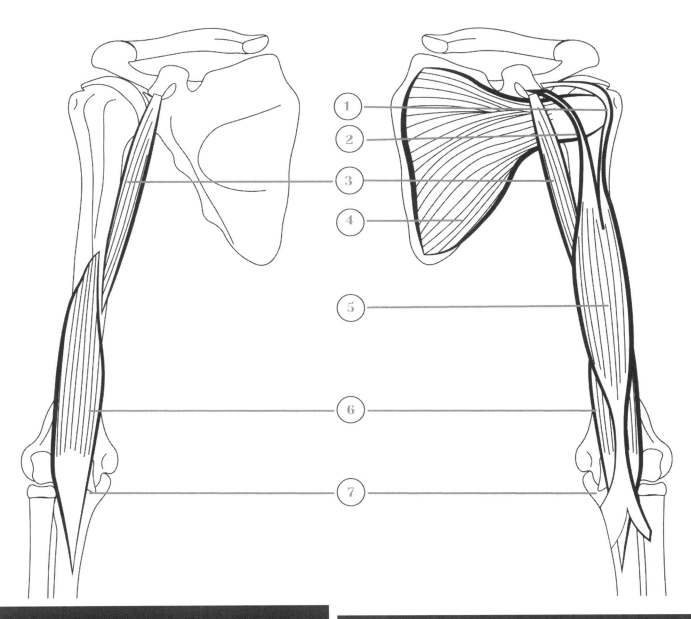

1. Long head (Biceps brachii)
2. Short head (Biceps brachii)
3. Coracobrachialis
4. Subscapularis (belongs to the Rotator cuff)
5. Biceps brachii
6. Brachialis
7. Ulna (proximal head)

NOTES

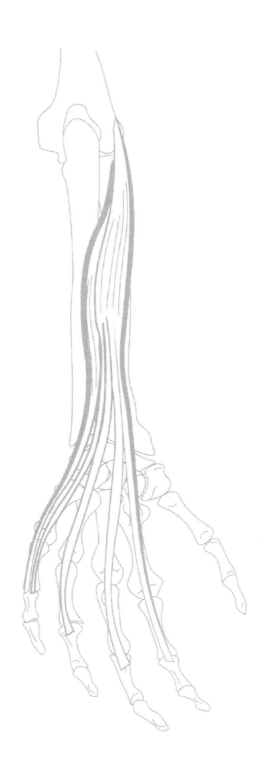

Muscles of the Arm (Posterior view)

UPPER LIMB

Rotator Cuff

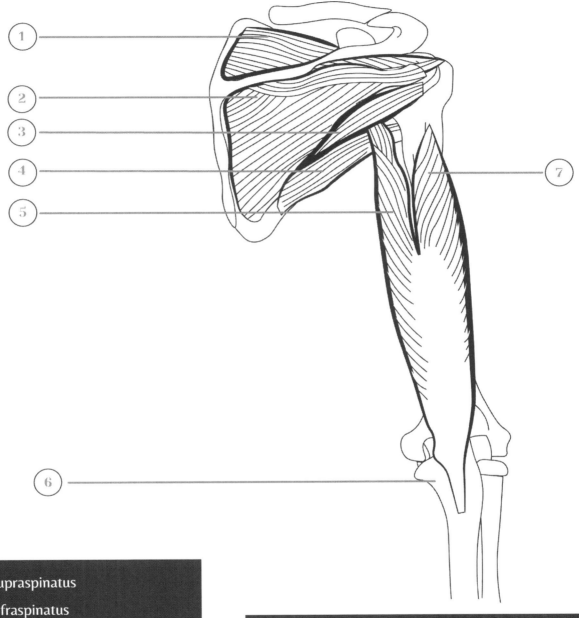

- 1. Supraspinatus
- 2. Infraspinatus
- 3. Teres minor
- 4. Teres major
- 5. Long head (Triceps brachii)
- 6. Ulna (proximal head)
- 7. Lateral head (Triceps brachii)

NOTES

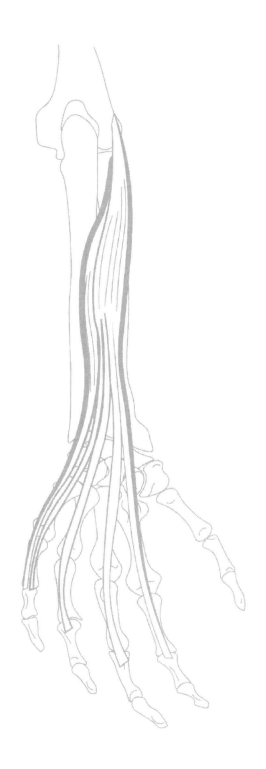

Muscles of the Forearm (Anterior View)

UPPER LIMB

1st Layer

2nd Layer

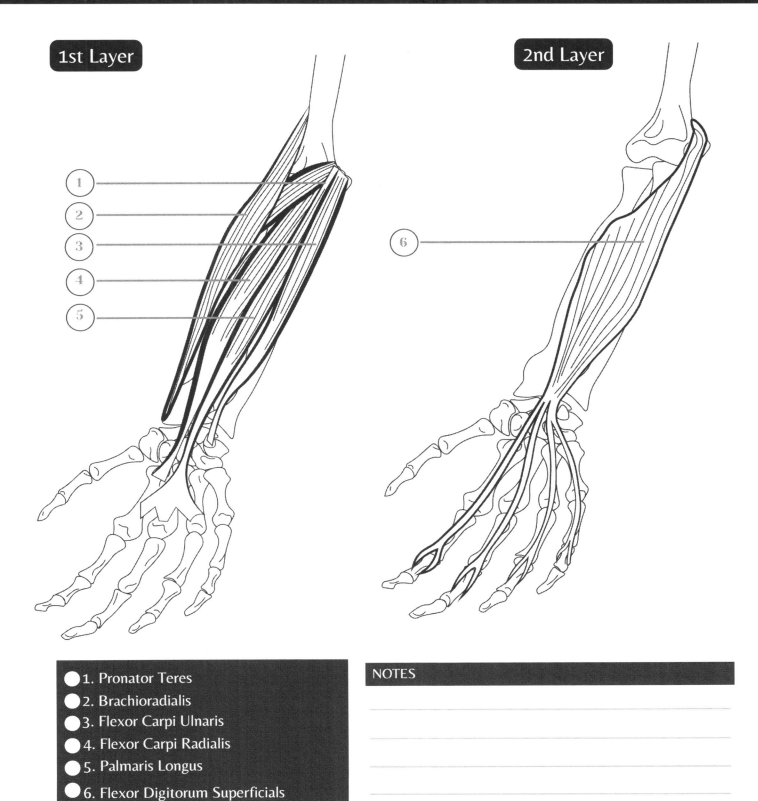

- 1. Pronator Teres
- 2. Brachioradialis
- 3. Flexor Carpi Ulnaris
- 4. Flexor Carpi Radialis
- 5. Palmaris Longus
- 6. Flexor Digitorum Superficals

NOTES

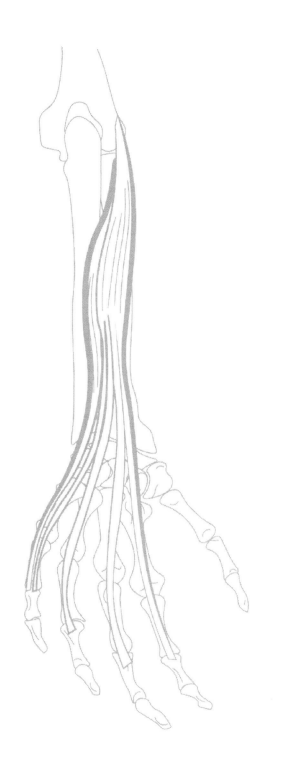

Muscles of the Forearm (Anterior View) — UPPER LIMB

3rd Layer
4th Layer

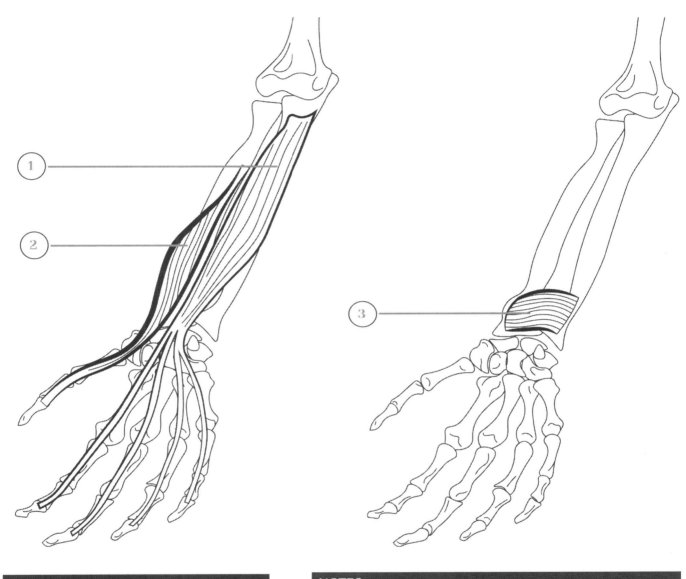

1. Flexor Digitorum Profundus
2. Flexor Pollicis Longus
3. Pronator Quadratus

NOTES

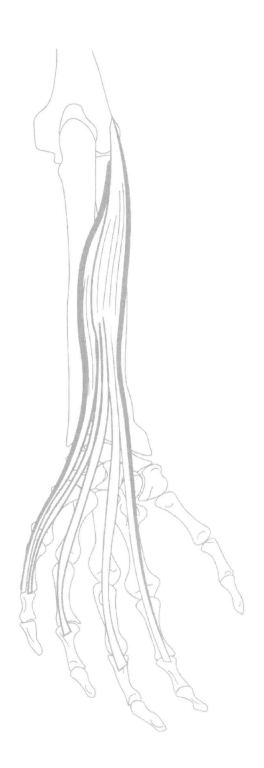

Muscles of the Forearm (Posterior View)

UPPER LIMB

Posterior view

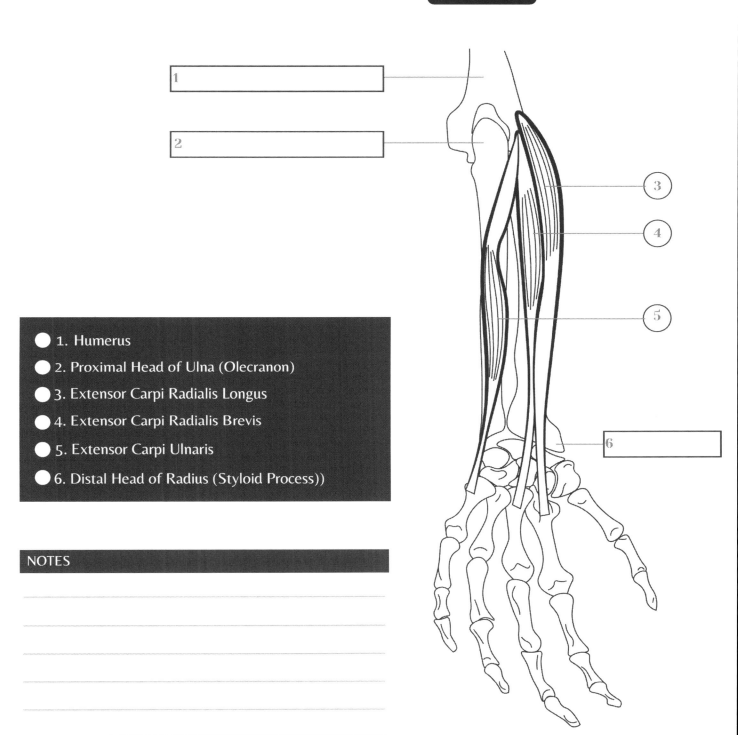

- 1. Humerus
- 2. Proximal Head of Ulna (Olecranon)
- 3. Extensor Carpi Radialis Longus
- 4. Extensor Carpi Radialis Brevis
- 5. Extensor Carpi Ulnaris
- 6. Distal Head of Radius (Styloid Process))

NOTES

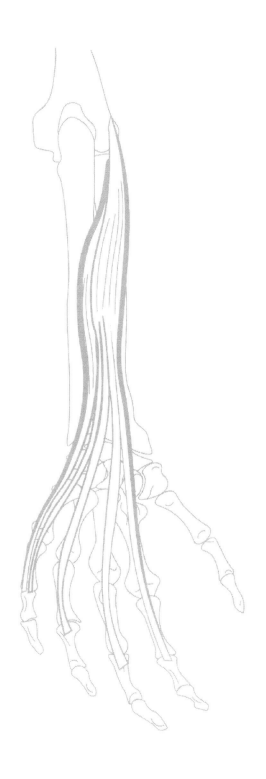

Muscles of the Forearm (Posterior View)

UPPER LIMB

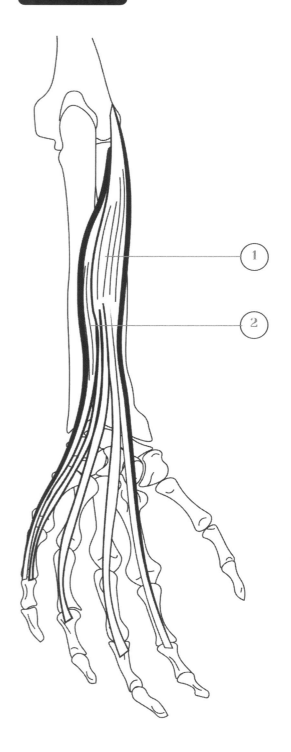

Posterior view

- 1. Extensor Digitorum
- 2. Extensor Digiti Minimi

NOTES

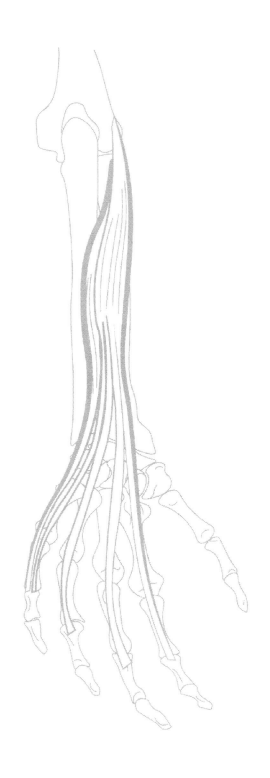

Muscles of the Forearm (Posterior View)

UPPER LIMB

Posterior view

1. Aconeus
2. Supinator
3. Abductor Pollicis Longus
4. Extensor Pollicis Longus
5. Extensor Pollicis Brevis
6. Extensor Indicis

NOTES

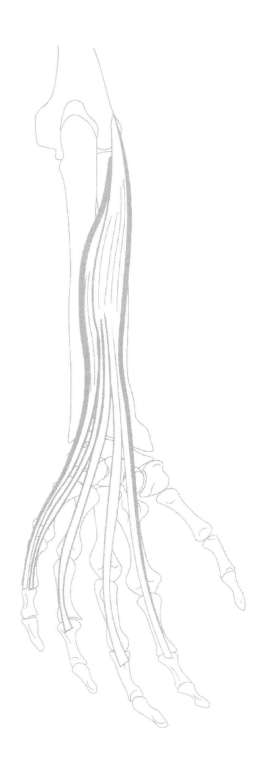

Arm Muscles - Review

UPPER LIMB

Anterior view

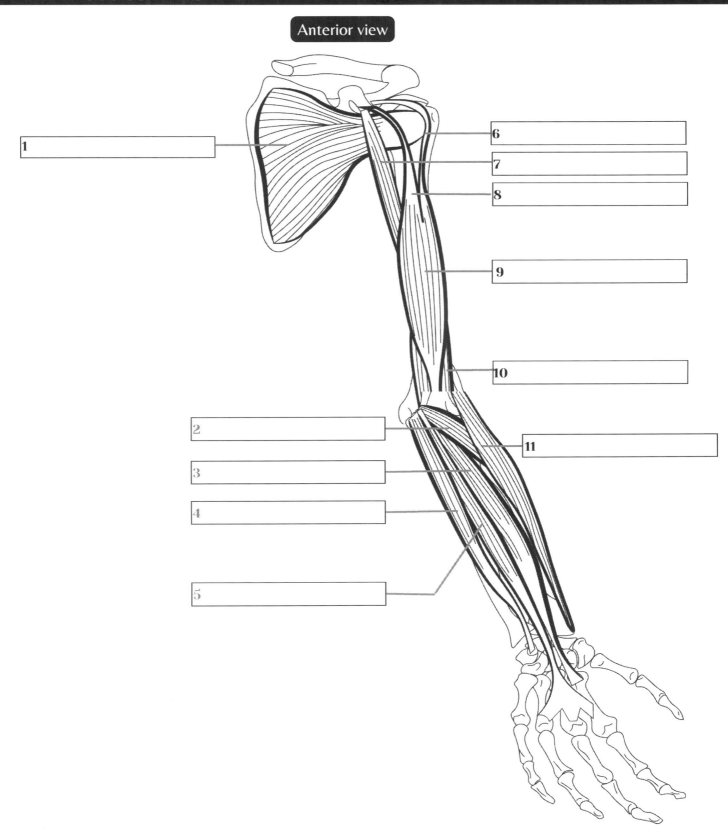

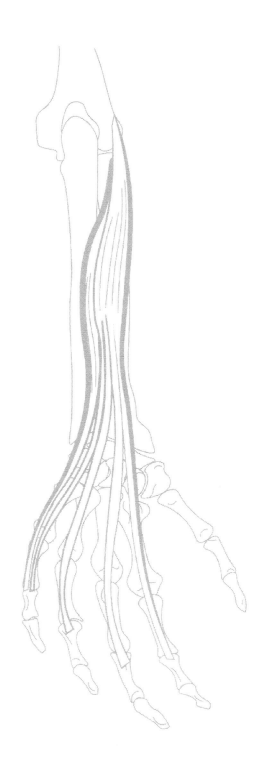

Hand - Review

UPPER LIMB

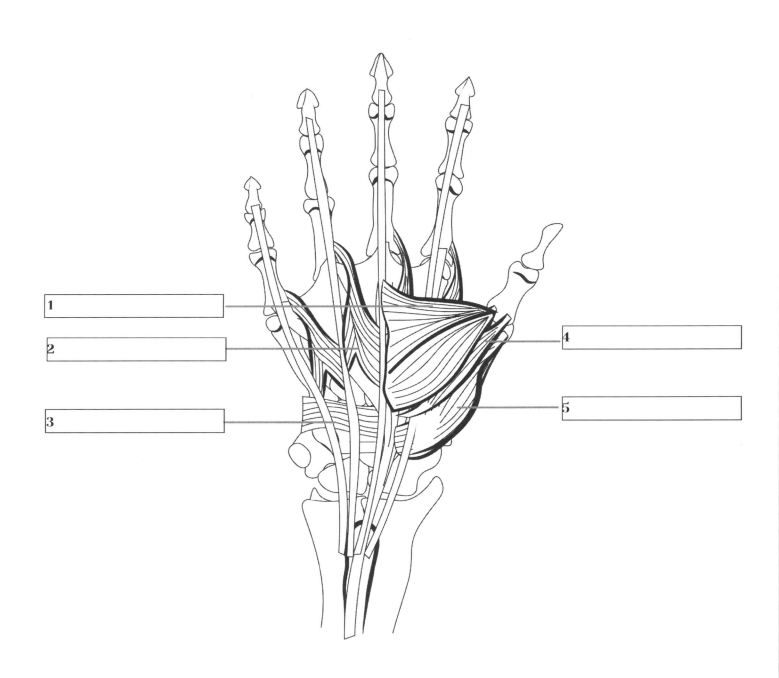

1.
2.
3.
4.
5.

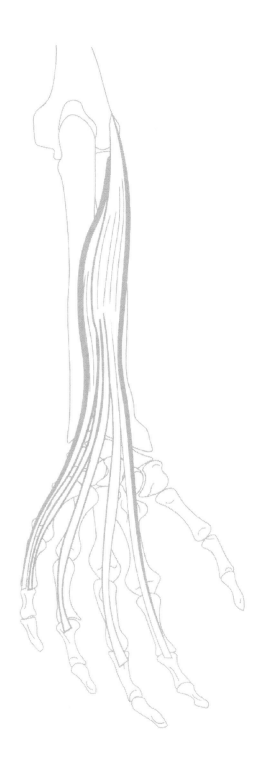

CHAPTER V

TRUNK

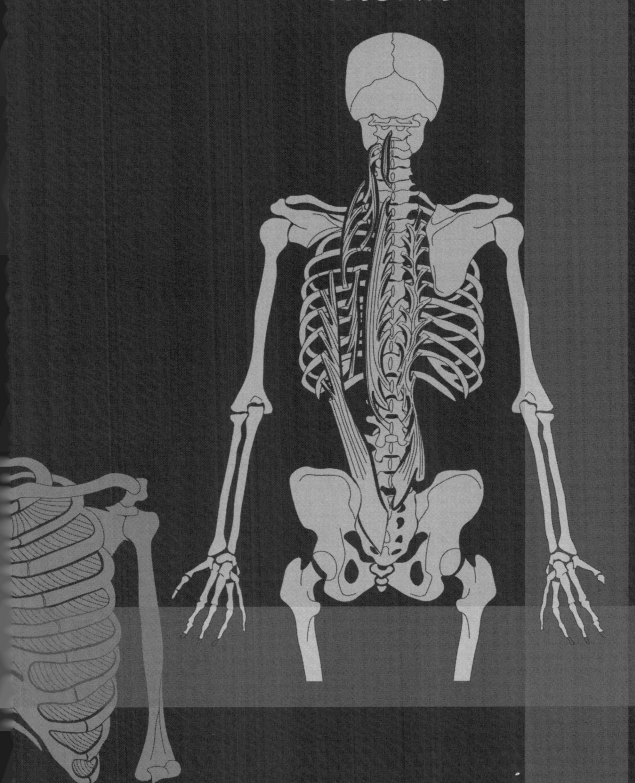

TRUNK

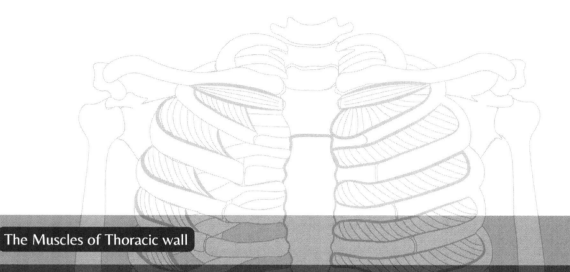

The Muscles of Thoracic wall

The 5 (five) major muscles include:

- Intercostales Externi (External Intercostal): Increases thoracic volume by drawing the ribs up during inspiration.
- Intercostales Interni (Internal Intercostal): Decreases thoracic volume by drawing the ribs downward during expiration.
- Transversus Thoracisc: Decreases the volume of the thoracic cavity by drawing down the ventral part of the ribs downward. during forceful expiration.
- Subcostales: Decreases thoracic volume by drawing down ribs during expiration.
- Innermost Intercostal: Increases thoracic volume by drawing the ribs down during inspiration.

Other muscles that are attached to the thoracic wall but are not apart of it includes:

- Serratus Anterior
- Pectoralis Major
- Pectoralis Minor
- Scalenus Muscles (Ant, Middle and Post.)

Ribcage Muscles — TRUNK

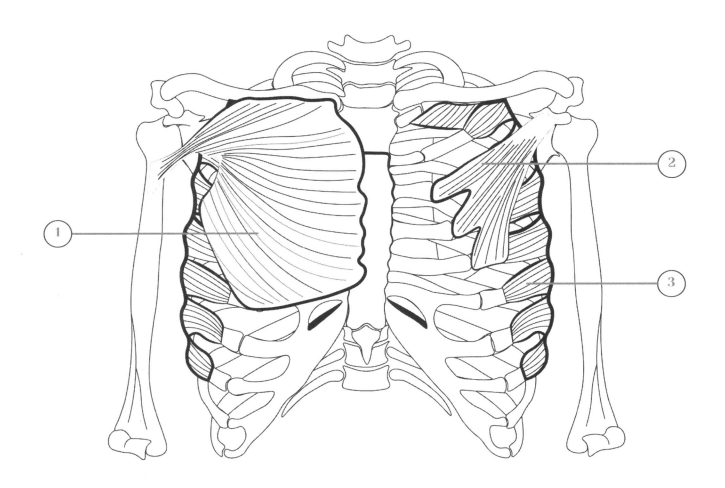

- 1. Pectoralis Major
- 2. Pectoralis Minor
- 3. Serratus Anterior

NOTES

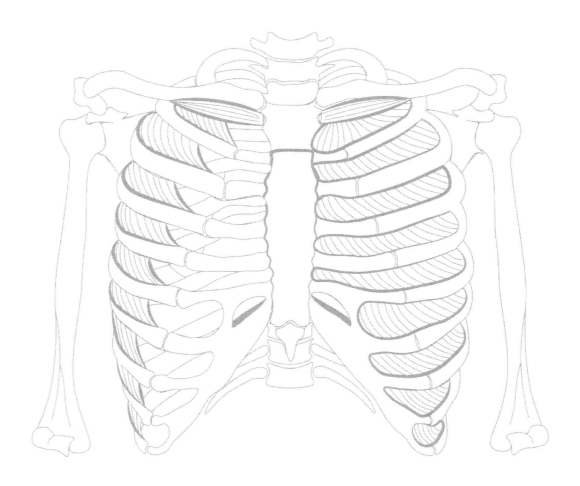

Ribcage Muscles — TRUNK

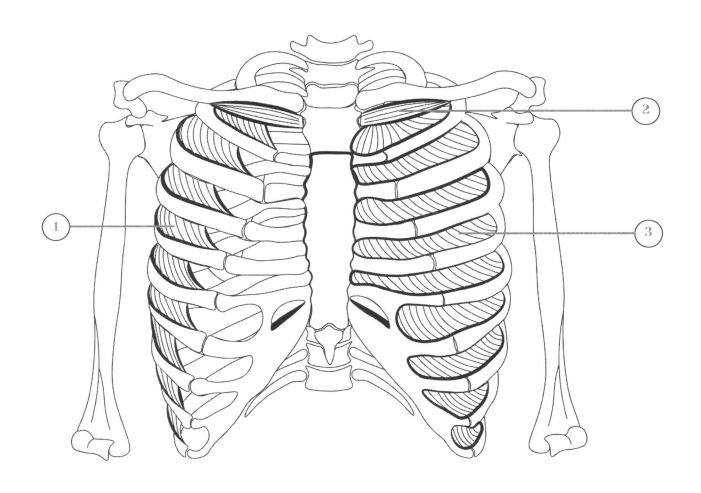

- 1. Intercostales Externi (External Intercostal)
- 2. Subclavius
- 3. Intercostales Interni (Internal Intercostal)

NOTES

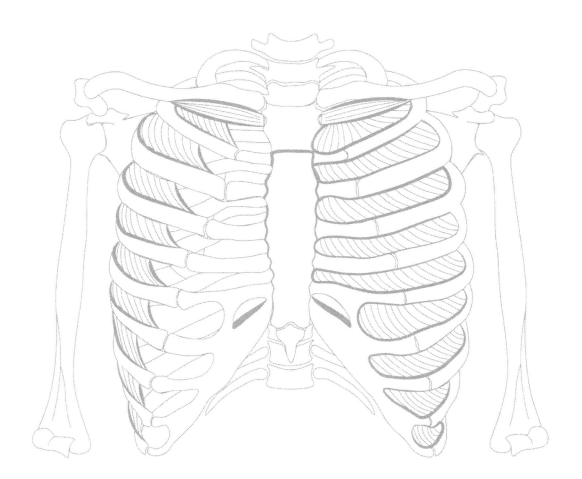

Ribcage Muscles

TRUNK

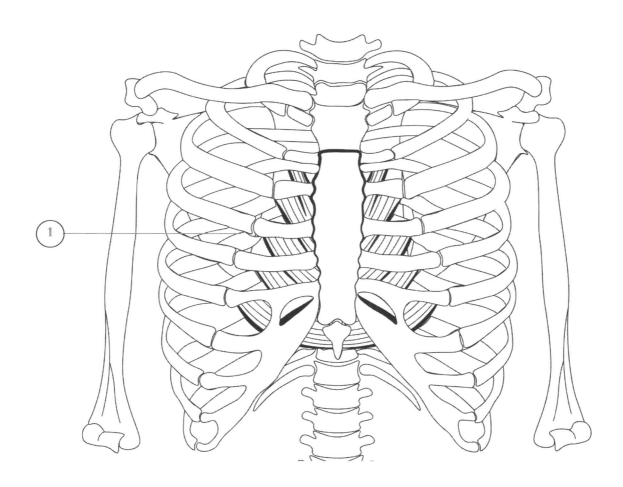

1. Transverse Thoracis

NOTES

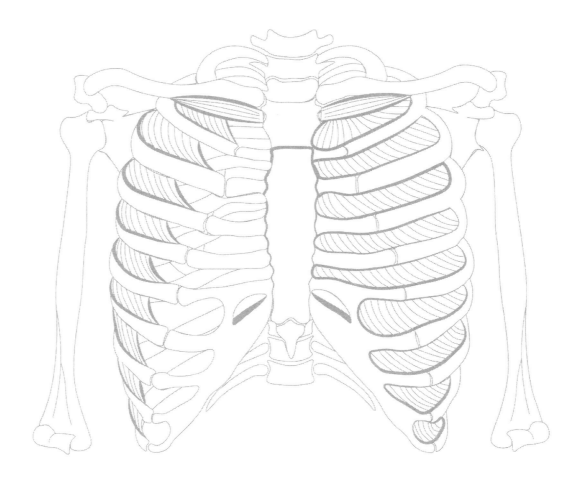

Ribcage Muscles

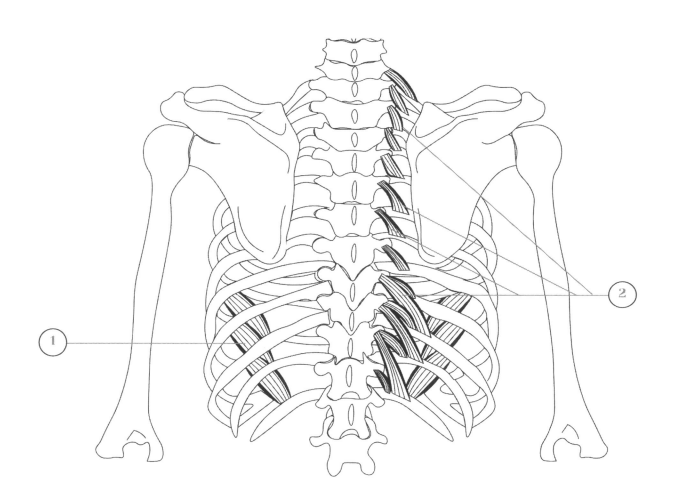

1. Subcostales
2. Levatores Costarum

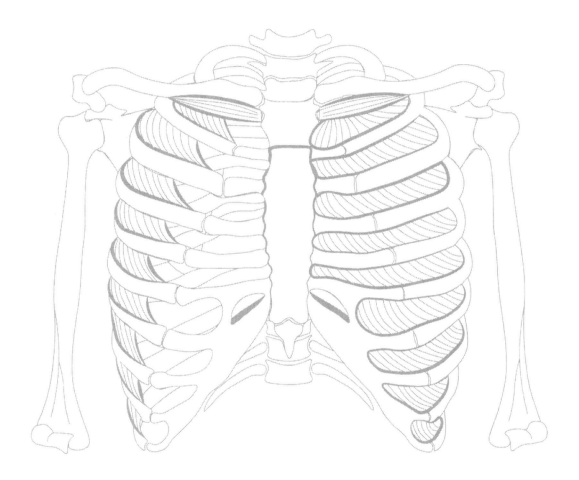

Intercostal Muscles Arrangement

TRUNK

Sagittal Section

Anterolateral view

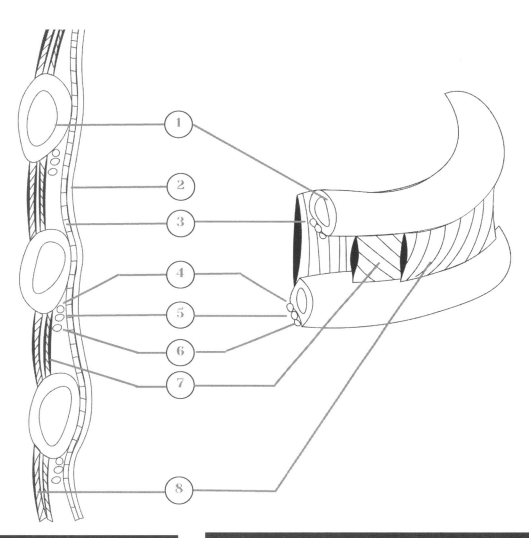

- 1. Rib (Section)
- 2. Parietal Pleura
- 3. Innermost Intercostal Muscle
- 4. Vein
- 5. Artery
- 6. Nerve
- 7. Intercostales Interni (Internal Intercostal)
- 8. Intercostales Externi (External Intercostal)

NOTES

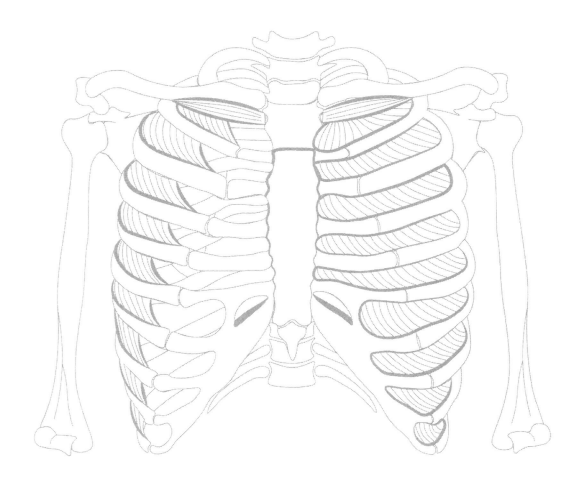

Diaphragm (Ribs removed)

TRUNK

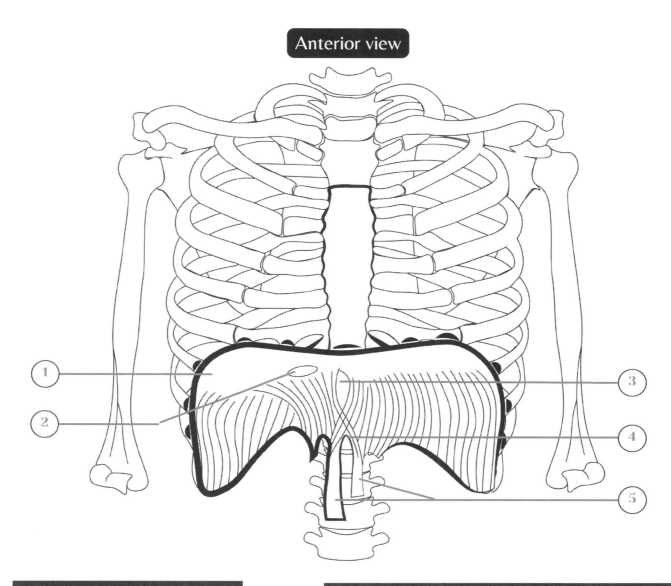

Anterior view

- 1. Diaphragm
- 2. Caval Hiatus
- 3. Oesophageal Hiatus
- 4. Aortic Hiatus
- 5. Vertebral Attachments

NOTES

Abdominal Muscles

TRUNK

Muscles of the Anterior Abdominal Wall

The 4 Main Abdominal Muscles

1. Rectus Abdominis
2. External Oblique
3. Internal Oblique
4. Transverse Abdominis

Abdominal Wall Layers Mnemonic : SSS EXITT

- S -Skin
- S -Subcutaneous Fat
- S -Superficial Fascia

- EX -External Oblique
- I   -Internal Oblique
- T   -Transverse Abdominis
- T   -Transversalis Fascia

Abdominal Muscles

TRUNK

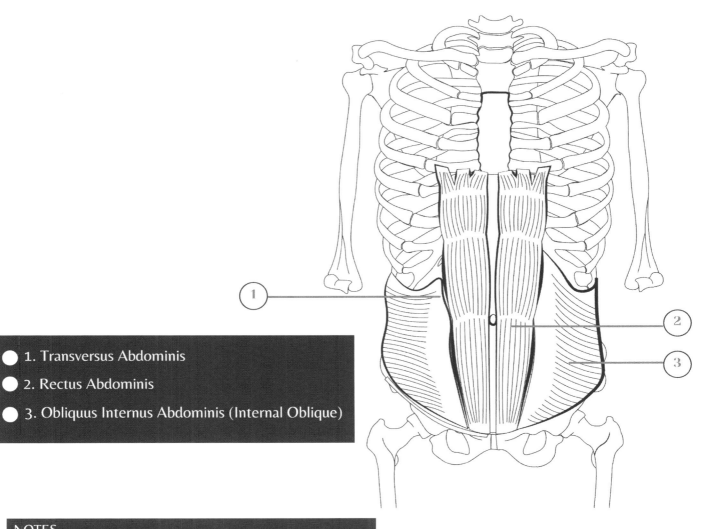

- 1. Transversus Abdominis
- 2. Rectus Abdominis
- 3. Obliquus Internus Abdominis (Internal Oblique)

NOTES

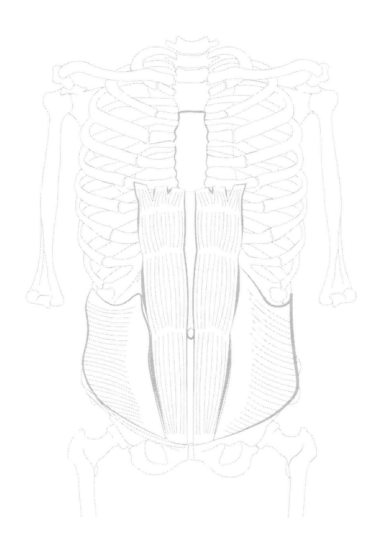

Abdominal Muscles (Axial section) TRUNK

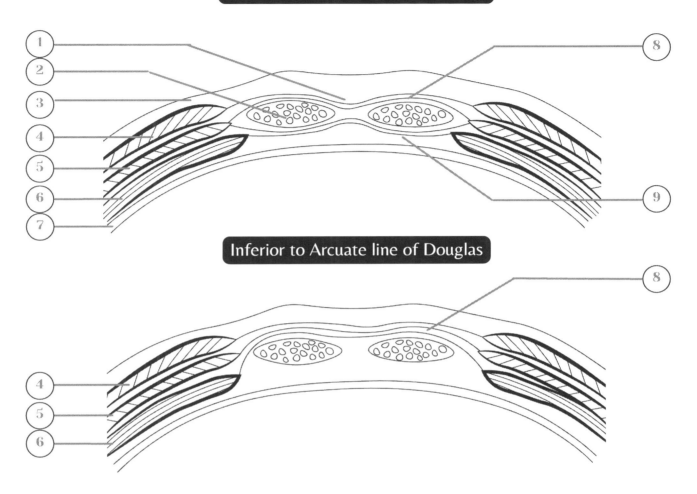

1. Linea Alba
2. Rectus Abdominis
3. Subcutaneous fatty tissue
4. Obliquus Externus Abdominis (External Oblique)
5. Obliquus Internus Abdominis (Internal Oblique)
6. Transversus Abdominis
7. Peritoneum
8. Rectus Sheath (Anterior Layer)
9. Rectus Sheath (Posterior Layer)

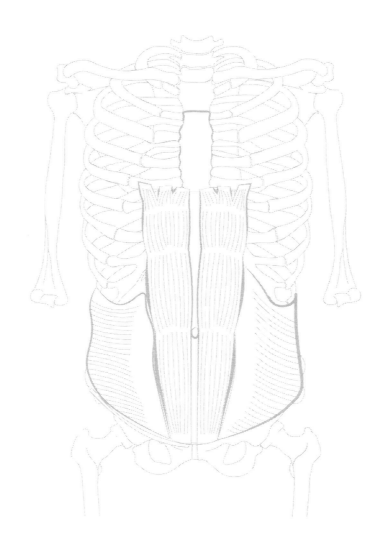

Abdominal Muscles

TRUNK

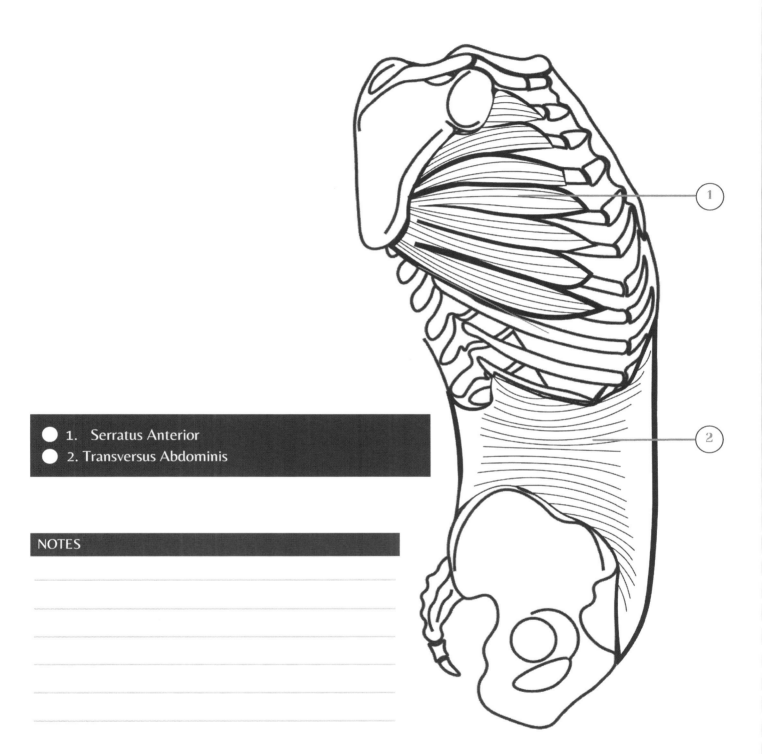

1. Serratus Anterior
2. Transversus Abdominis

NOTES

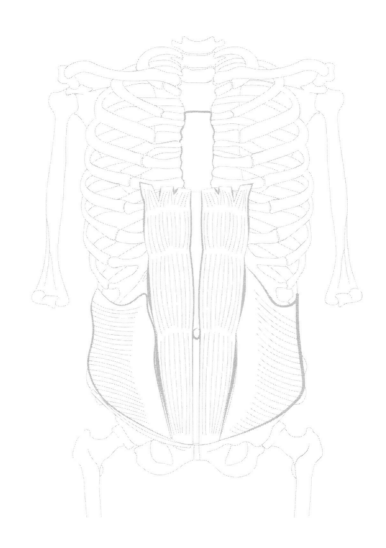

Abdominal Muscles

TRUNK

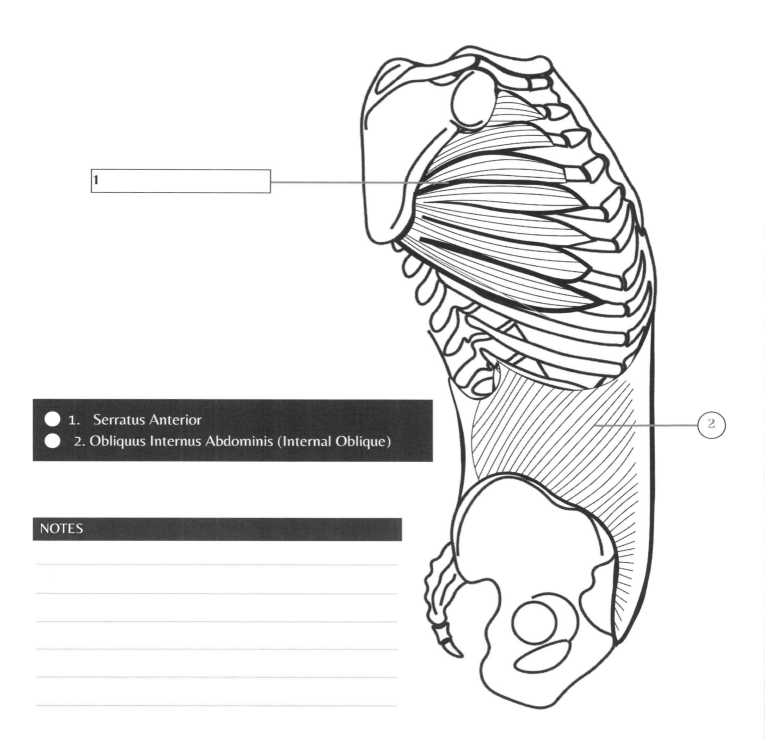

1. Serratus Anterior
2. Obliquus Internus Abdominis (Internal Oblique)

NOTES

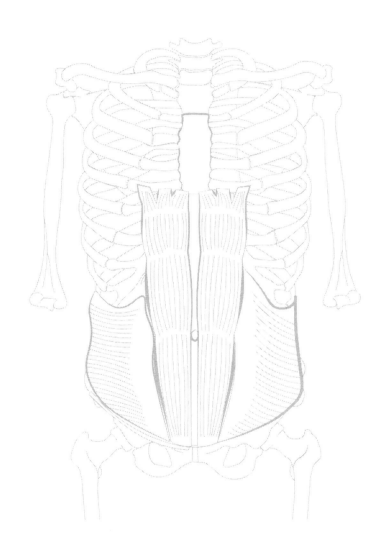

Abdominal Muscles

TRUNK

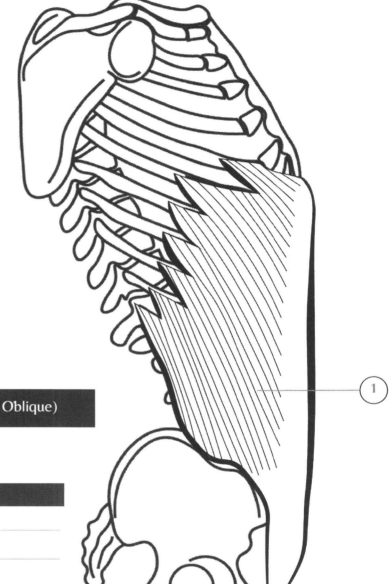

● 2. Obliquus Externus Abdominis (External Oblique)

NOTES

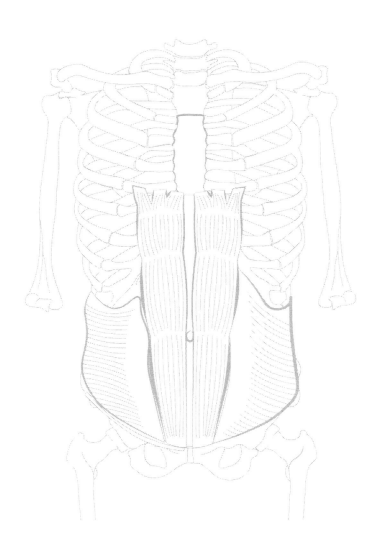

Trunk Muscles - Review

TRUNK

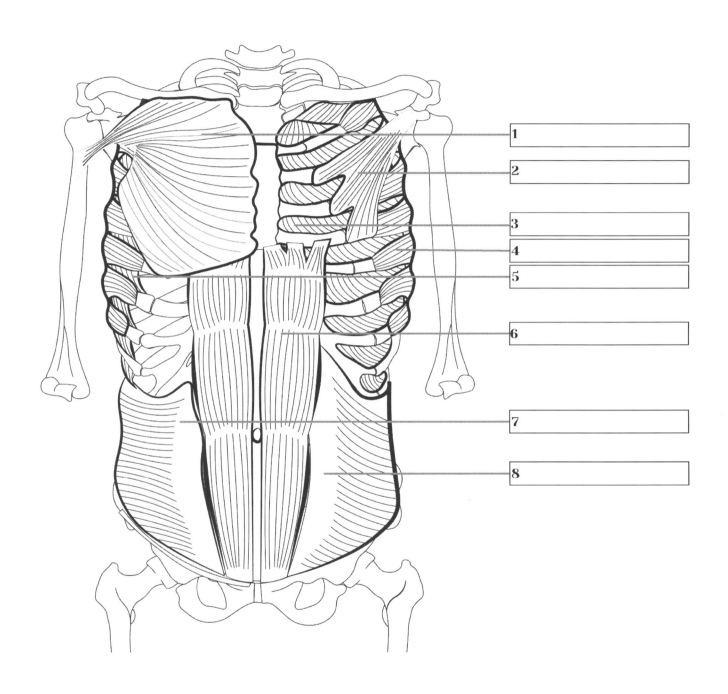

1.
2.
3.
4.
5.
6.
7.
8.

TRUNK

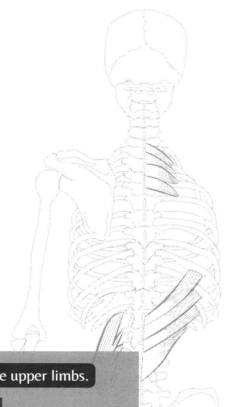

Muscles of the back that act on the upper limbs.

First Layer

- Trapezius
- Latissimus Dorsi

Second Layer

- Levator Scapulae
- Rhomboid Minor
- Rhomboid Major

Muscles of the Back (Superficial Layers) TRUNK

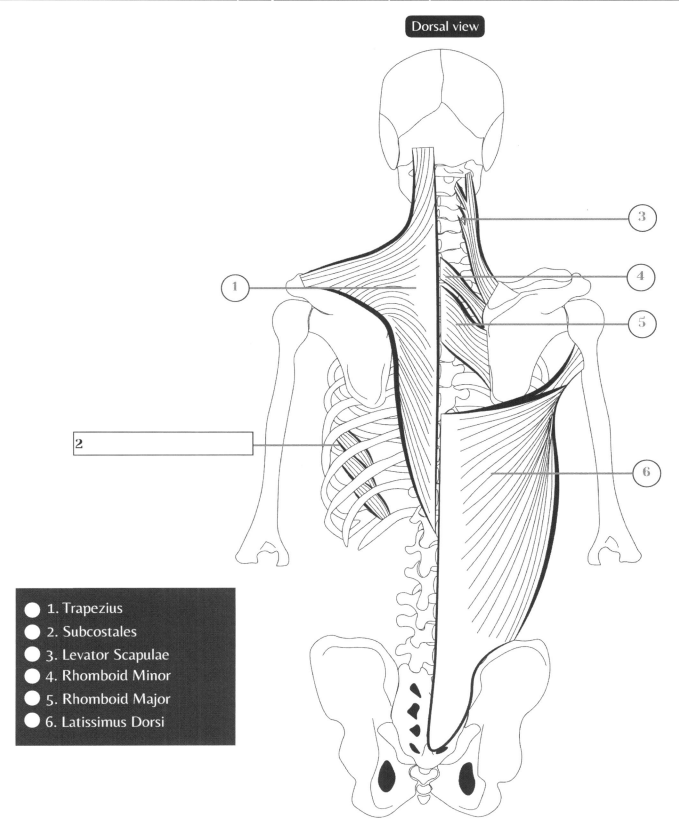

- 1. Trapezius
- 2. Subcostales
- 3. Levator Scapulae
- 4. Rhomboid Minor
- 5. Rhomboid Major
- 6. Latissimus Dorsi

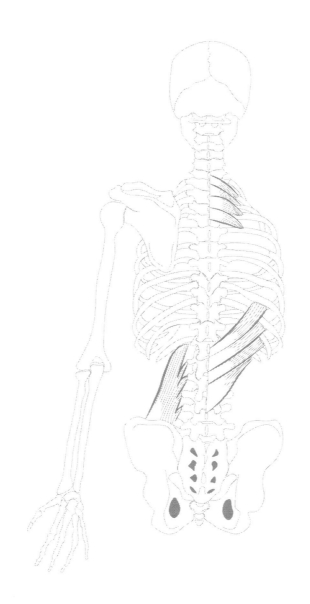

Muscles of the Back (Deep Layers)

TRUNK

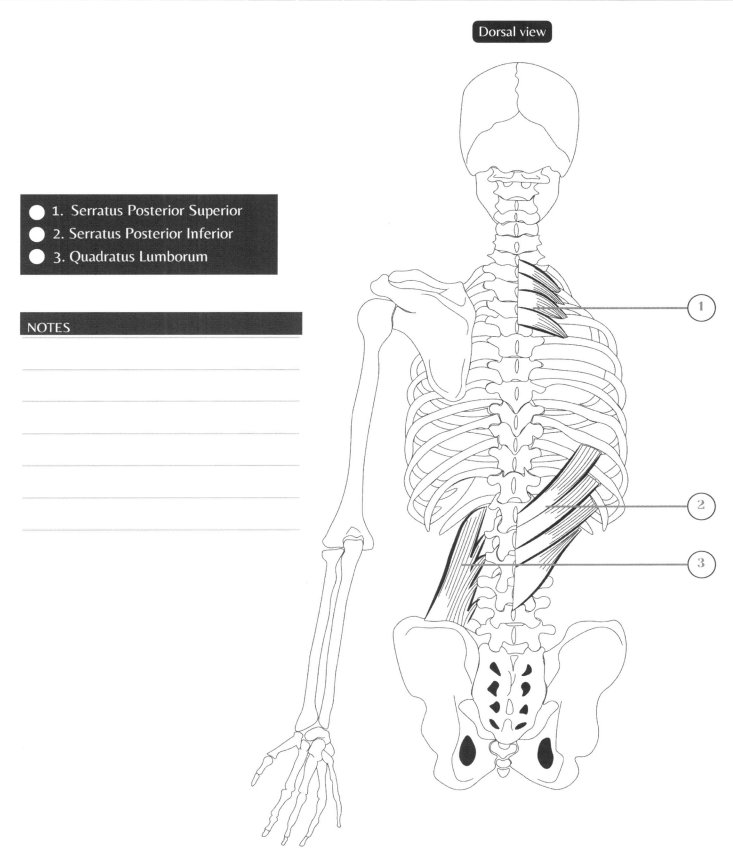

Dorsal view

1. Serratus Posterior Superior
2. Serratus Posterior Inferior
3. Quadratus Lumborum

NOTES

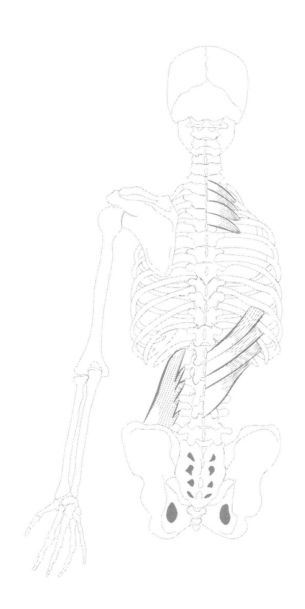

Muscles of the Back (Deep Layers)

TRUNK

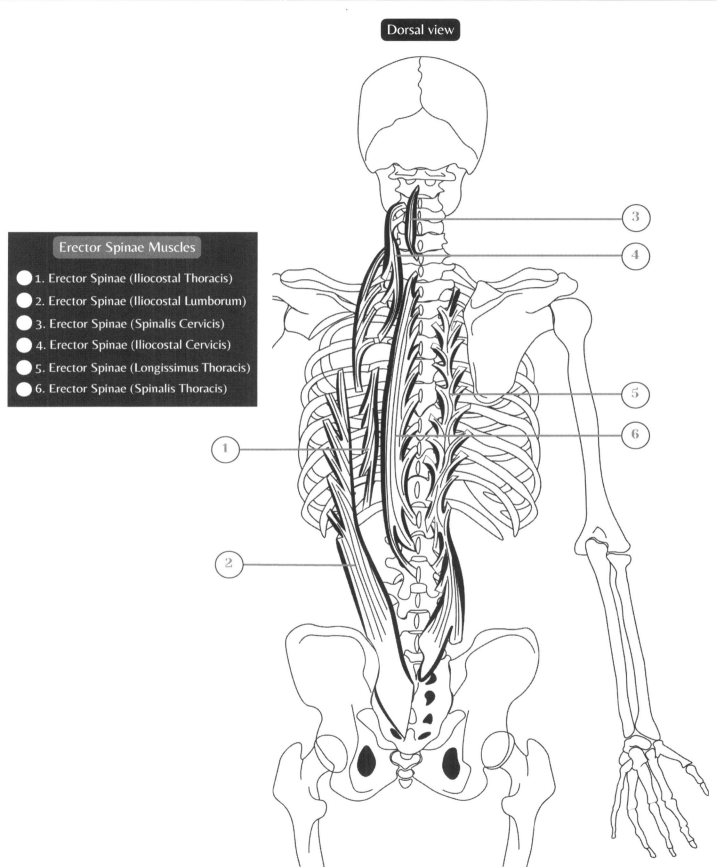

Dorsal view

Erector Spinae Muscles

- 1. Erector Spinae (Iliocostal Thoracis)
- 2. Erector Spinae (Iliocostal Lumborum)
- 3. Erector Spinae (Spinalis Cervicis)
- 4. Erector Spinae (Iliocostal Cervicis)
- 5. Erector Spinae (Longissimus Thoracis)
- 6. Erector Spinae (Spinalis Thoracis)

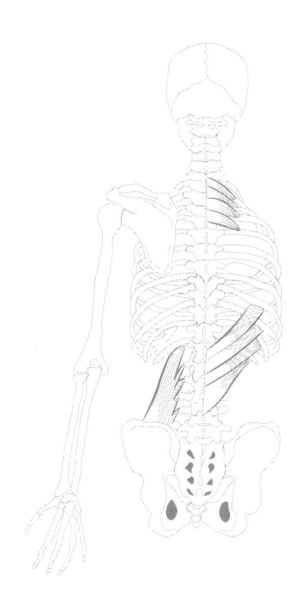

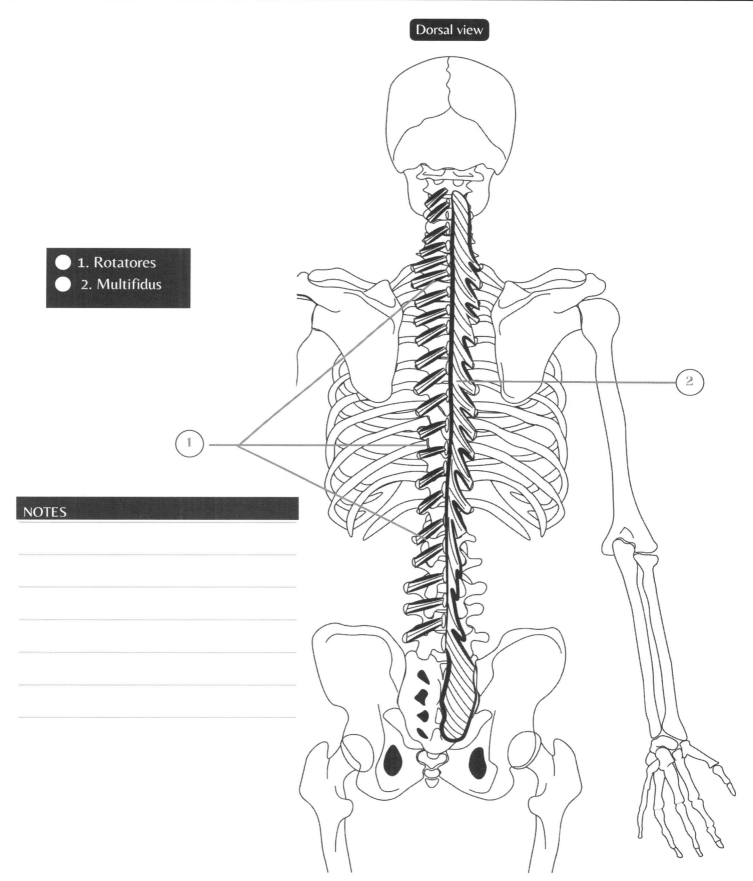

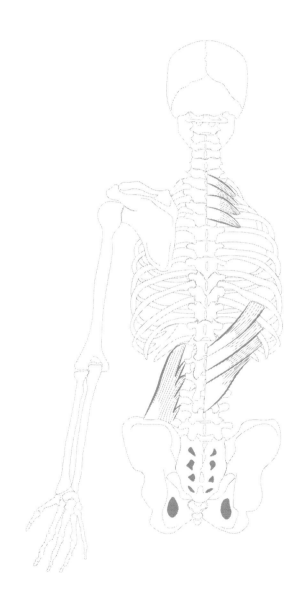

Muscles of the Back (Deep Layers)

TRUNK

Dorsal view

- 1. Transversospinalis (Semispinalis Capitis)
- 2. Quadratus Lumborum
- 3. Intertransversarii
- 4. Interspinalis

NOTES

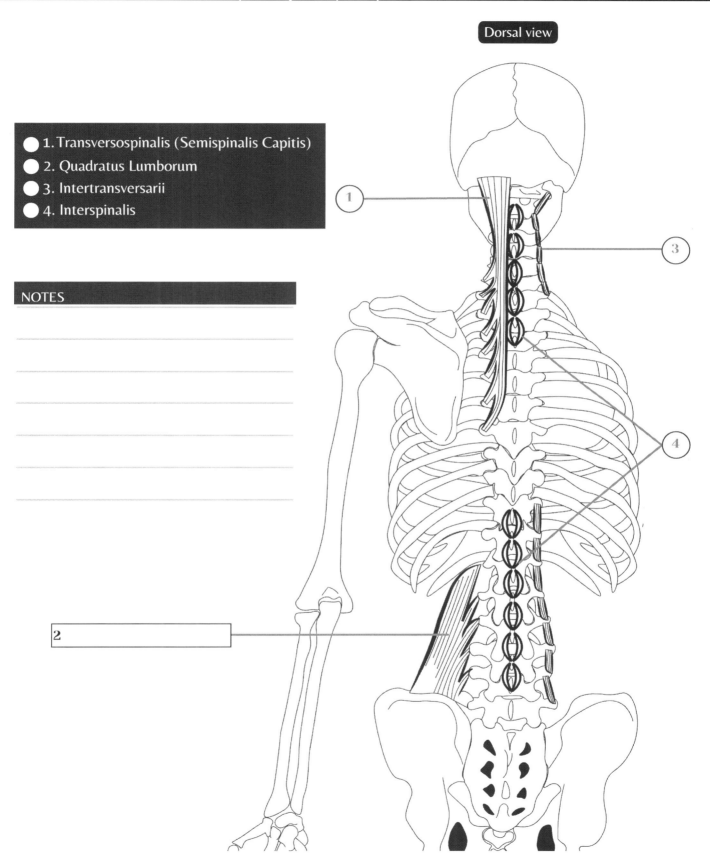

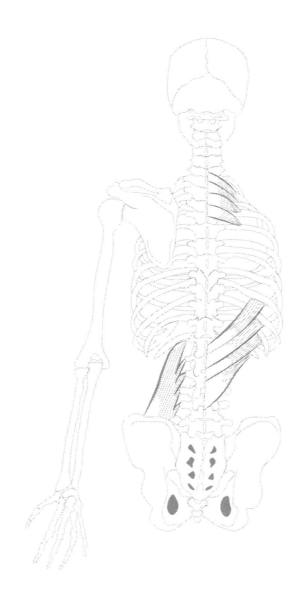

Muscles of the Back - Review TRUNK

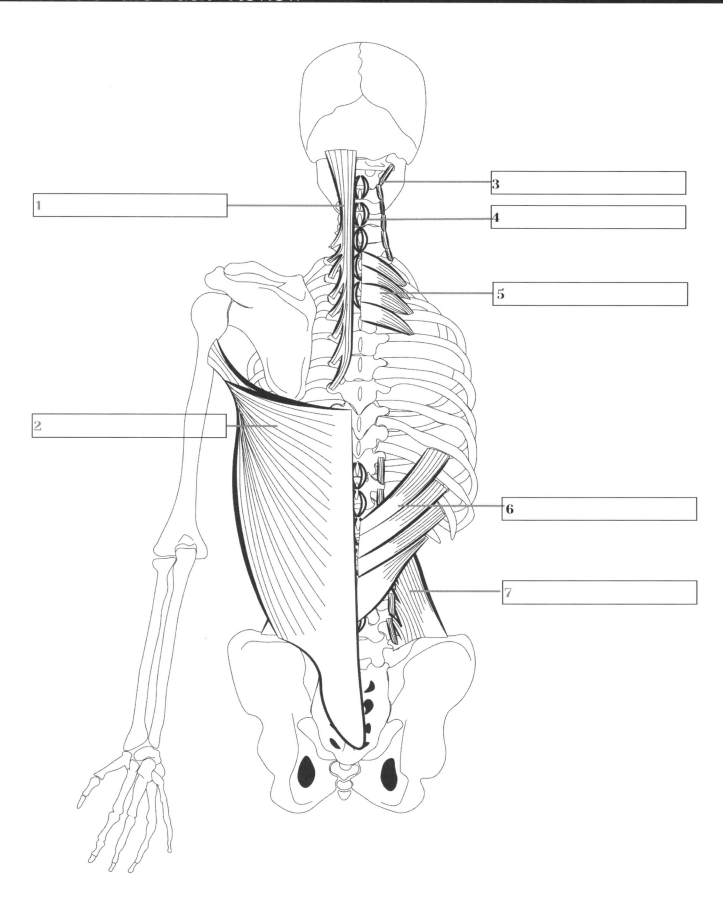

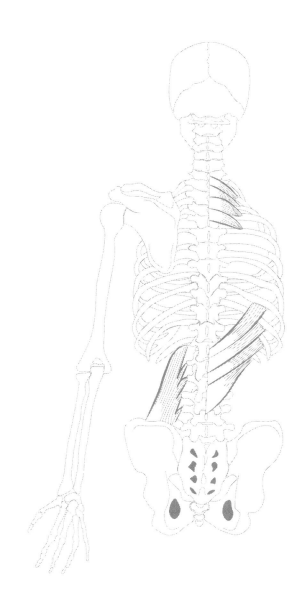

CHAPTER VI
HIP & LOWER LIMB

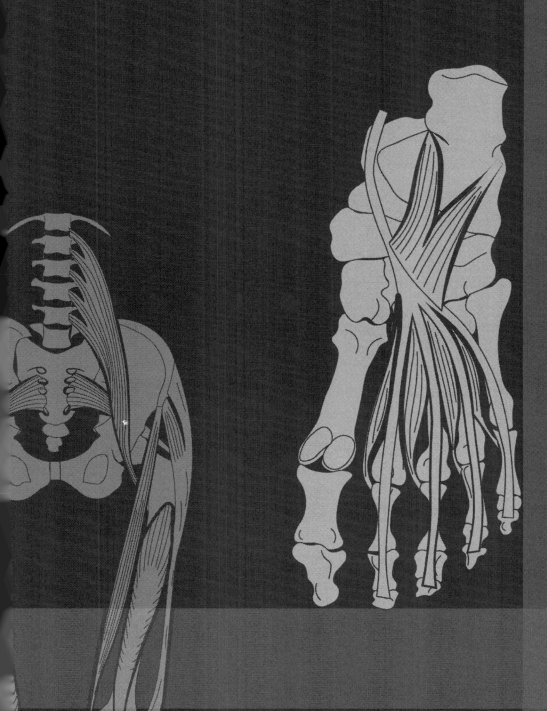

HIP & LOWER LIMB

The Muscles of the hip and thigh

These muscles can be divided into three main groups:

- Iliopsoas group
- Gluteal muscles
- Hip adductors

Iliopsoas group

- Iliacus
- Psoas major
- Psoas minor

Superficial Gluteal muscles:

- Gluteus Maximus
- Gluteus Medius
- Gluteus Minimus
- Tensor Fasciae Latae

Deep Gluteal muscles:

- Piriformis
- Gemellus superior
- Gemellus inferior
- Obturator internus
- Obturator externus
- Quadratus femoris

Hip adductors

- Gracilis
- Pectineus
- Adductor Magnus
- Adductor Longus
- Adductor Brevis
- Adductor Minimus

Thigh Flexors

HIP & LOWER LIMB

Anterior view

- 1. Psoas Major (Part of Iliopsoas)
- 2. Tensor Fasciae latae
- 3. Sartorius
- 4. Vastus intermedius (Quadriceps femoris)
- 5. Iliacus (Part of Iliopsoas)
- 6. Inguinal ligament
- 7. Rectus femoris (Quadriceps femoris)
- 8. Vastus lateralis (Quadriceps femoris)
- 9. Vastus Medialis (Quadriceps femoris)

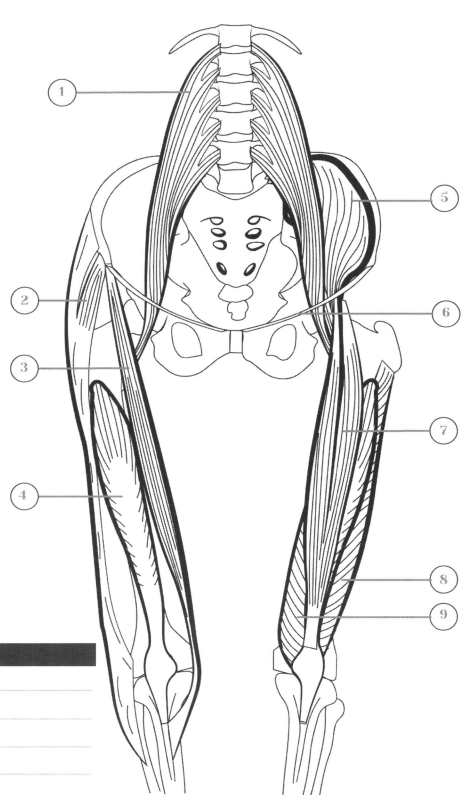

NOTES

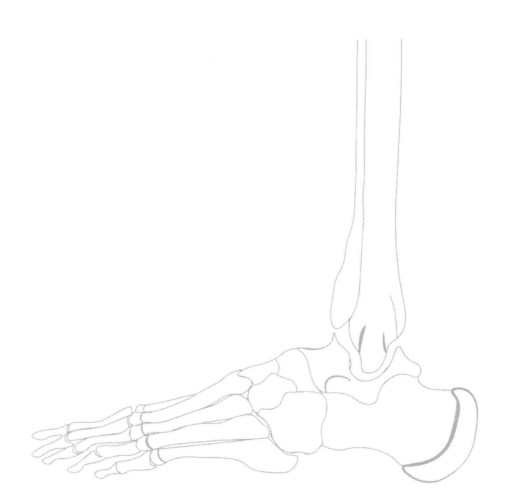

Thigh Adductors

HIP & LOWER LIMB

Anterior view

- 1. Piriformis
- 2. Pectineus
- 3. Adductor brevis
- 4. Adductor longus
- 5. Gracilis
- 6. Adductor magnus

NOTES

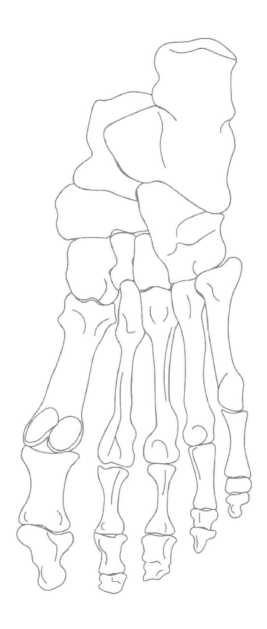

Thigh Adductors
HIP & LOWER LIMB

Posterior view

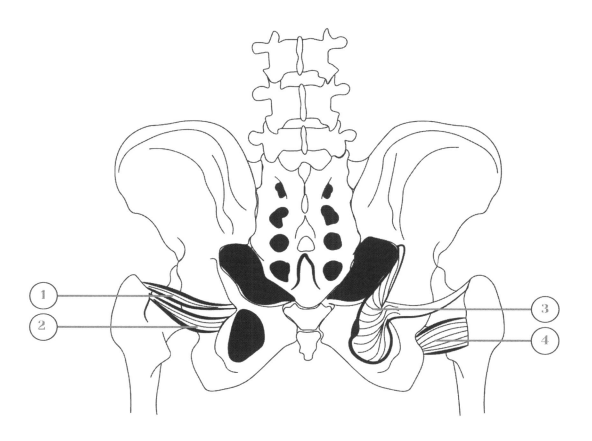

- 1. Gemellus Superior
- 2. Gemellus Inferior
- 3. Quadratus Internus
- 4. Quadratus Femoris

NOTES

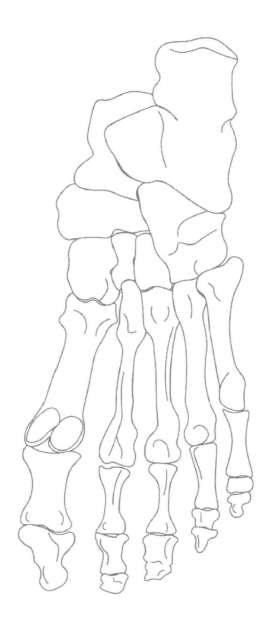

Thigh Adductors

HIP & LOWER LIMB

Posterior view

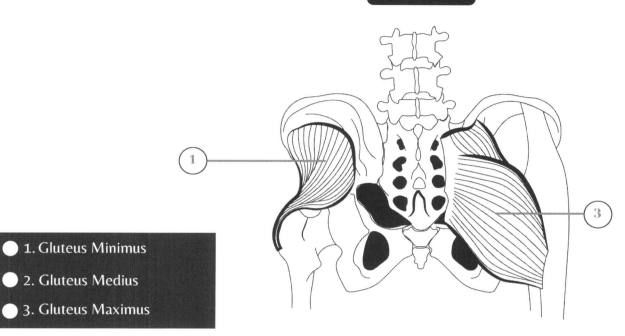

- 1. Gluteus Minimus
- 2. Gluteus Medius
- 3. Gluteus Maximus

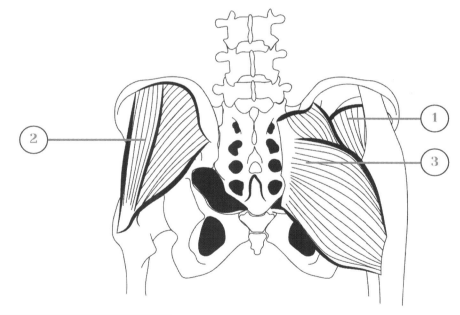

NOTES

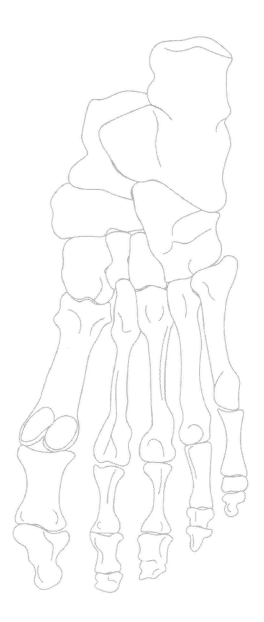

Hamstring Muscles

HIP & LOWER LIMB

Posterior view

- 1. Quadratus Femoris
- 2. Biceps Femoris
- 3. Semimembranosus
- 4. Semitendinosus

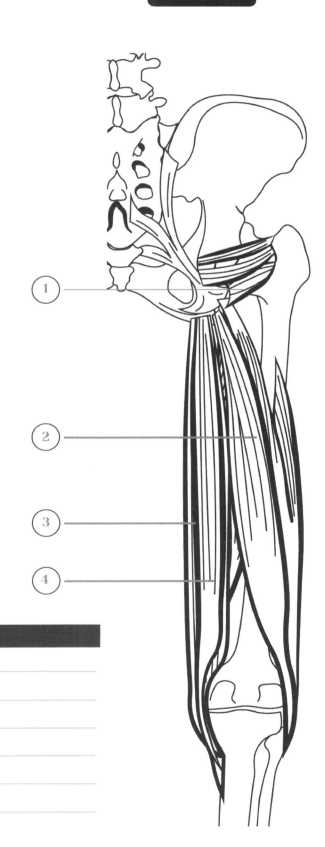

NOTES

Muscles of the Foot

The muscles of the leg are divided into three (3) compartments:

Anterior compartment

- Anterior Tibialis: Inverts and Dorsiflexes the foot.
- Extensor Hallucis Longus: Dorsiflexes the foot and extends the big toe.
- Extensor Digitorum Longus: Dorsiflexes the foot and extends the 4 lateral toes.
- Peroneus Tertius: Dorsiflexes and Everts the foot.

Lateral compartment

- Peroneus Longus: Eversion of the foot.
- Peroneus Brevis: Eversion of the foot.

Posterior compartment

- Gastrocnemius: Plantar flexes the foot.
- Soleus: Plantar flexes the foot.
- Plantaris: Plantar flexes the foot.

Leg Muscles

HIP & LOWER LIMB

Anterolateral view

- 1. Extensor Digitorum Longus
- 2. Peroneus Longus
- 3. Extensor Hallucis Longus

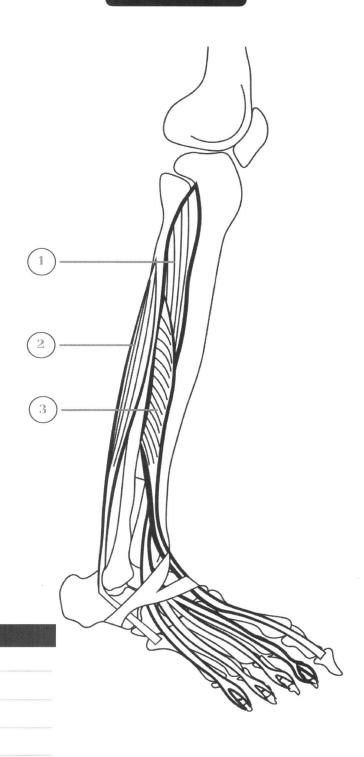

NOTES

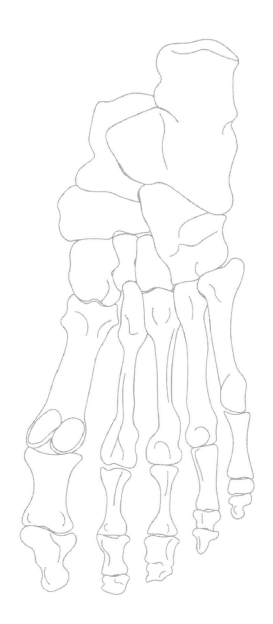

Leg Muscles

HIP & LOWER LIMB

Anterolateral view

- 1. Extensor Digitorum Longus
- 2. Gastrocnemius
- 3. Peroneus Longus
- 4. Extensor Hallucis Longus
- 5. Tibialis Anterior
- 6. Peroneus Tertius
- 7. Inferior Extensor Retinaculum

NOTES

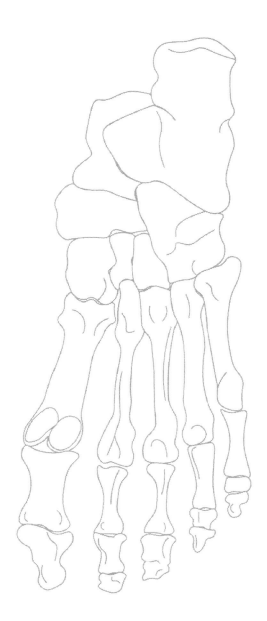

Muscles of the Calf

HIP & LOWER LIMB

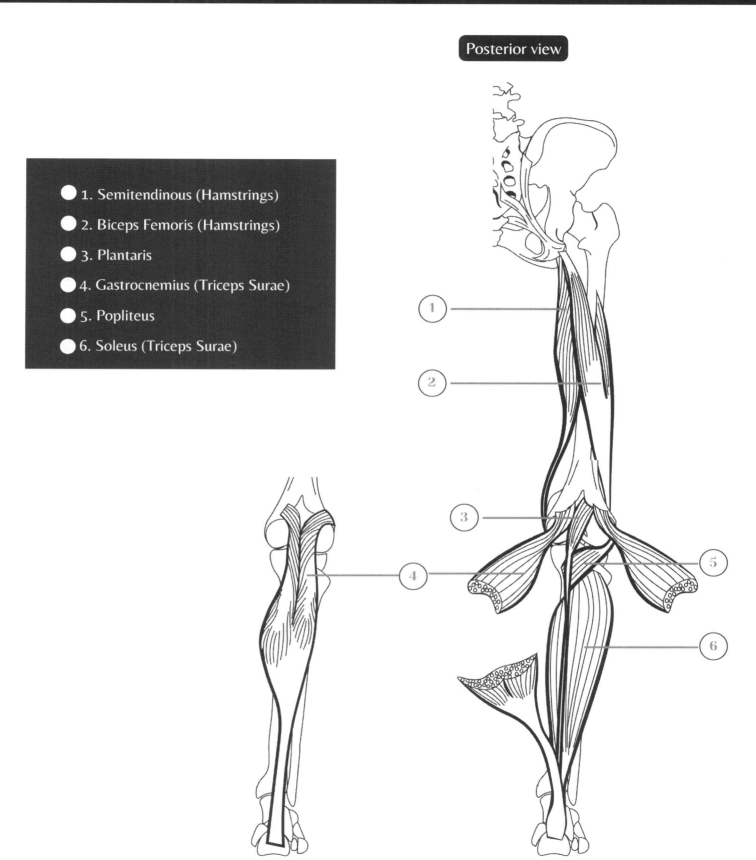

Posterior view

- 1. Semitendinous (Hamstrings)
- 2. Biceps Femoris (Hamstrings)
- 3. Plantaris
- 4. Gastrocnemius (Triceps Surae)
- 5. Popliteus
- 6. Soleus (Triceps Surae)

Muscles of the Foot

These muscles are Intrinsic muscles.

First Layer

- Abductor Hallucis: Abducts and flexes the great toe.
- Flexor Digitorum Brevis: Flexes the lateral four toes.
- Abductor Digiti Minimi: Abducts and flexes the 5th digit (pinky toe).

Second Layer

- Quadratus Plantae: Assists the flexor digitorum longus in flexing the lateral 4 toes.
- Lumbricals: Flexes at the base of the toes but also extends the end of the toes.

Third Layer

- Flexor Hallucis Brevis: Flexes the great toe.
- Adductor Hallucis: Adducts the great toe and assists in forming the transverse arch of the foot.
- Flexor Digiti Minimi Brevis: Flexes the 5th digit (pinky toe).

Fourth Layer

- Plantar Interossei: Adducts digits 3-5 and flexes those toes.
- Dorsal interossei: Abducts digits 2-4 and flexes those toes.

Muscles of the Foot (First Layer)

HIP & LOWER LIMB

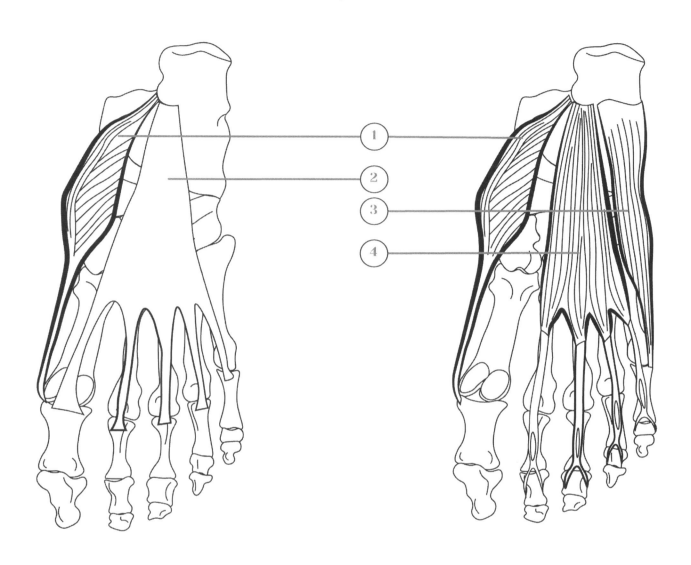

- 1. Abductor Hallucis
- 2. Plantar aponeurosis
- 3. Abductor Digiti Minimi
- 4. Flexor Digitorum Brevis

NOTES

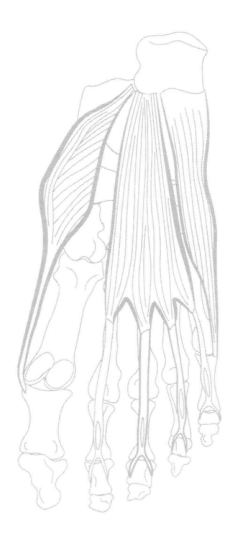

Muscles of the Foot

HIP & LOWER LIMB

Second layer (Plantar view)

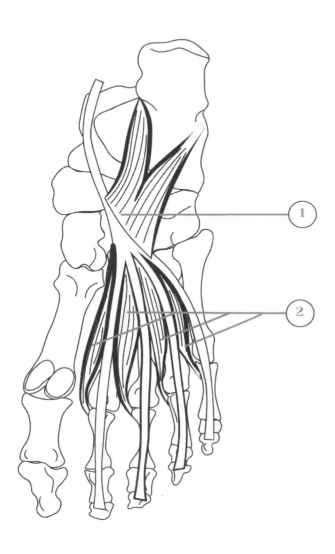

Third layer (Plantar view)

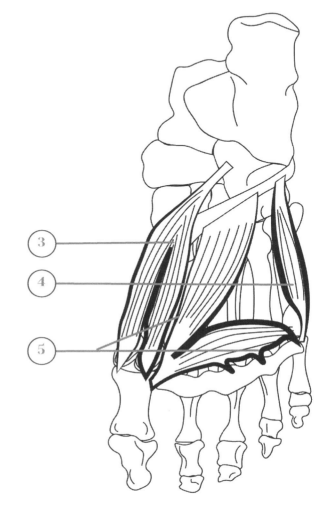

- 1. Quadratus Plantae
- 2. Lumbricales
- 3. Flexor Hallucis Brevis
- 4. Flexor Digiti Minimi Brevis
- 5. Abductor Hallucis

NOTES

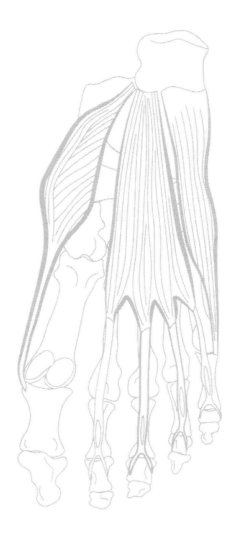

Muscles of the Foot (Fourth Layer)

HIP & LOWER LIMB

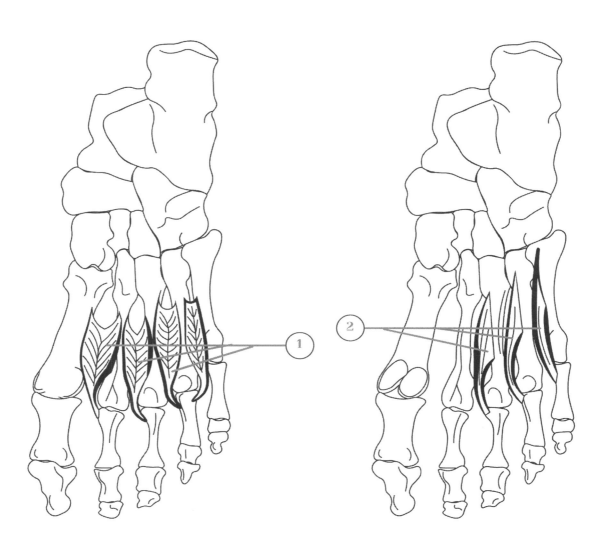

- 1. Dorsal Interossei
- 2. Plantar Interossei

NOTES

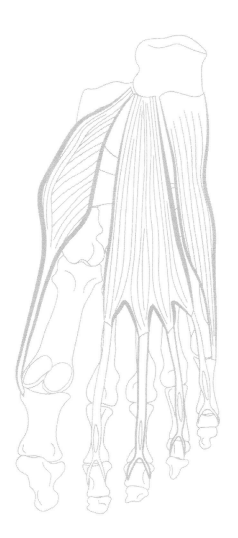

Foot - lateral view

HIP & LOWER LIMB

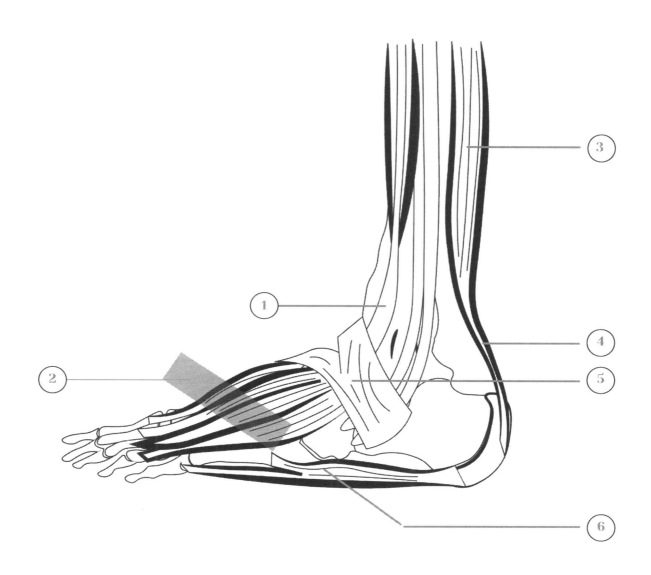

- 1. Extensor Digitorum Longus (Tendon)
- 2. Extensor Digitorum Brevis
- 3. Gastrocnemius
- 4. Achilles Tendon
- 5. Inferior Extensor Retinaculum
- 6. Abductor Hallucis

NOTES

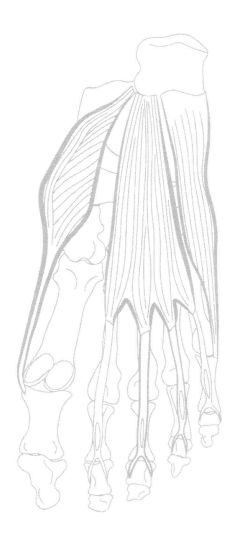

Lower Limb - Review

HIP & LOWER LIMB

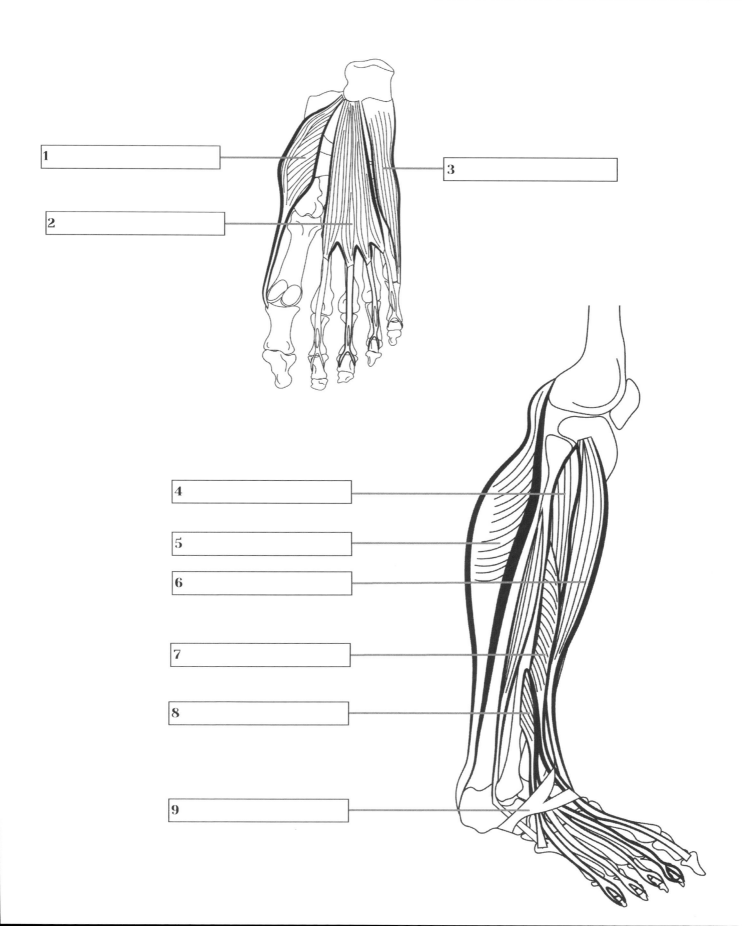

1. _____
2. _____
3. _____
4. _____
5. _____
6. _____
7. _____
8. _____
9. _____

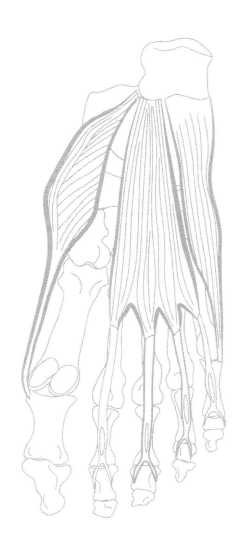

OTHER BOOKS FROM THE MEDICAL NOTES SERIES

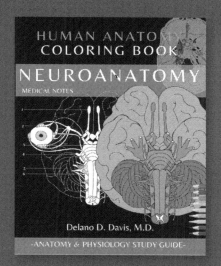
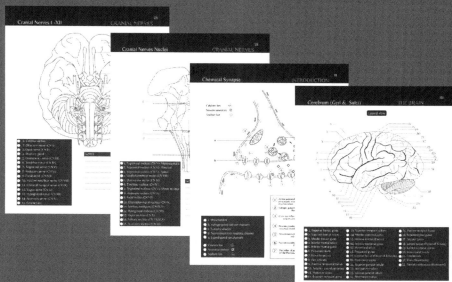

- Detailed neuroanatomical diagrams
- Gross anatomy & physiology
- High yield summaries and overviews
- Add & personalize your notes
- Chapter reviews and self-tests
- Access to video tutorials & quizzes

Scan QR code to purchase →

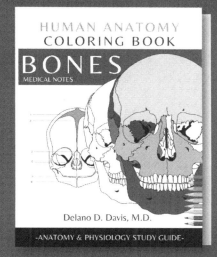
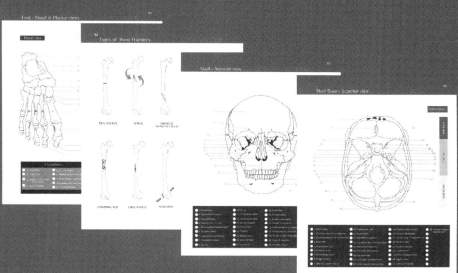

- Detailed diagrams of the bones of the skeletal system
- Mnemonics to remember bones
- High yield summaries and overviews
- Add & personalize your notes
- Long bone fractures
- Chapter reviews and self-tests
- Access to video tutorials & quizzes

Scan QR code to purchase →

MEDICAL ESSENTIALS +
MEDICAL EDUCATION THE EASY WAY

If you enjoy and found this book helpful, please help us by rating and, or leaving a positive review of this book on Amazon. Thank you.

Connect with us:

Follow us on all our social media platforms

MEDICAL ESSENTIALS PLUS

For questions and customer service;

Send us an email at medicalessentialsplus@gmail.com
Follow Us on Instagram @ medicalessentialsplus
Subscribe to our Youtube channel " Medical Essentials Plus"
for tutorials and Quizzes.

Made in the USA
Columbia, SC
05 December 2024

48547385R00089